Obstetric Emergencies

Managing Obstetric Emergencies

C. Cox
FRCS (Ed) FRCOG
Consultant Obstetrician and Gynaecologist,
New Cross Hospital, Wolverhampton WV10 0QP, UK

K. Grady
BSc FRCA
Consultant Anaesthetist,
South Manchester University Hospitals' NHS Trust,
Southmoor Road, Manchester M23 9LT, UK

CONSULTANT EDITOR

R.B. Johanson
MA BSc MD MRCOG
Consultant Obstetrician and Gynaecologist,
North Staffordshire Hospital NHS Trust, Newcastle Road,
Stoke-on-Trent ST4 6QG, UK

© BIOS Scientific Publishers Limited, 1999

First published 1999
Reprinted 2002

A CIP catalogue record for this book is available from the British Library.

ISBN 1 85996 122 3

1 0 0 2 8 5 7 2 2 9

BIOS Scientific Publishers Ltd
9 Newtec Place, Magdalen Road, Oxford OX4 1RE, UK
Tel. +44 (0)1865 726286. Fax +44 (0)1865 246823
World Wide Web home page: http://www.bios.co.uk/

Important Note from the Publisher
The information contained within this book was obtained by BIOS Scientific Publishers Ltd from sources believed by us to be reliable. However, while every effort has been made to ensure its accuracy, no responsibility for loss or injury whatsoever occasioned to any person acting or refraining from action as a result of information contained herein can be accepted by the authors or publishers.

The reader should remember that medicine is a constantly evolving science and while the authors and publishers have ensured that all dosages, applications and practices are based on current indications, there may be specific practices which differ between communities. You should always follow the guidelines laid down by the manufacturers of specific products and the relevant authorities in the country in which you are practising.

Production Editor: Jonathan Gunning.
Typeset by J&L Composition Ltd, Filey, UK.
Printed by T.J. International Ltd, Padstow, UK.

CONTENTS

3. MEDICAL EMERGENCIES

4. LEGAL ISSUES

CONTRIBUTORS

Khaled, MA MB BS LMSSA MRCOG
Specialist Registrar, Department of Obstetrics and Gynaecology, Hope Hospital, Stott Lane, Salford M6 8HD, UK

Maguire, S MB ChB
Specialist Registrar, Department of Anaesthesia, Hope Hospital, Stott Lane, Salford M6 8HD, UK

O'Donnell, E MRCOG Dip.Med.Ed. DCH
Consultant Obstetrician and Gynaecologist, Manor Hospital, Walsall, West Midlands WS11 9PS, UK

Saad, MEF MB BS DGO FAMS FRCOG
Associate Professor, Department of Obstetrics and Gynaecology, Faculty of Medicine – University of Khartoum, PO Box 102, Khartoum, Sudan

Thomas, E DM MRCOG DA
Specialist Registrar in Obstetrics and Gynaecology, New Cross Hospital, Wolverhampton WV10 0QP, UK

Wasson, C BSc MB ChB FRCA
Specialist Registrar, Department of Anaesthesia, Manchester Royal Infirmary, Oxford Road, Manchester M13 9WL, UK

ABBREVIATIONS

ABGs	arterial blood gases
ACE	angiotensin converting enzyme
AED	automatic external defibrillator
ALS	advanced life support
APTT	activated partial thromboplastin time
ARDS	adult respiratory distress syndrome
ARF	acute renal failure
ARM	artificial rupture of membranes
AV	atrioventricular
AVPU	alert, responsive to voice, responsive to pain, unresponsive
BP	blood pressure
CCU	coronary care unit
CPAP	continuous positive airways pressure
CPR	cardiopulmonary resuscitation
CTG	cardiotocograph
CVP	central venous pressure
CXR	chest X-ray
DIC	disseminated intravascular coagulation
DKA	diabetic ketoacidosis
DVT	deep vein thrombosis
ECG	electrocardiogram
ECV	external cephalic version
EMD	electromechanical dissociation
FAST	focused abdominal sonography in trauma
FBC	full blood count
FDPs	fibrin degradation products
FFP	fresh frozen plasma
FH	fetal heart
G&S	group and save serum
GCS	Glasgow Coma Scale
GKI	glucose, potassium, insulin
HDU	high dependency unit
i.v.i.	intravenous infusion
ICU	intensive care unit
JVP	jugular venous pressure
LFTs	liver function tests
MIST	mechanism, injuries, symptoms and signs, treatment
MRI	magnetic resonance imaging
MSSU	midstream specimen of urine
NIBP	non-invasive blood pressure
NMDA	N-methyl-D-aspartate
PCWP	pulmonary capillary wedge pressure
PEEP	positive end expiratory pressure
PEFR	peak expiratory flow rate
PIH	pregnancy-induced hypertension
RAST	radioallergosorbent test
RR	respiratory rate
RUQ	right upper quadrant
SaO$_2$	arterial oxygen saturation

SCBU	special care baby unit
SHO	senior house officer
SpR	Specialist Registrar
U&Es	urea and electrolytes
U/O	urine output
V/Q	ventilation/perfusion
VF/VT	ventricular fibrillation/ventricular tachycardia

PREFACE

This book is intended for those in the front line of acute obstetric care on the delivery suite, including consultant obstetricians, obstetricians-in-training, anaesthetists with a commitment to obstetrics, midwives and all team members responsible for the care of the pregnant woman. Life-threatening obstetric emergencies occur infrequently and when they do, are not managed well. Many consultant obstetricians do not come across conditions such as uterine inversion or shoulder dystocia on a regular or even occasional basis and the opportunity to teach the acute management of such cases is limited. A didactic approach to the management of these and other life-threatening obstetric emergencies has been adopted so that in the emergency situation clear instructions are provided. There may be alternative methods but these are safe and effective.

This book is not intended to replace teaching on the labour ward, practical obstetric skills courses or larger texts. It does, however, provide a framework and backup to such teaching. It is hoped that it will act as a basis for regular obstetric 'fire drills', to be practised as part of a multidisciplinary approach as suggested in *Towards Safer Childbirth*.

In the era of evidence-based medicine, it is essential that good evidence is used to modify clinical experience and support decisions about the management of individual patients (bearing in mind their wishes as well). Unfortunately, our practice is limited by availability of high quality research data. Accordingly, much of the evidence summarized in this book is not based on randomized controlled trials. Using the established hierarchy system, 'next best' evidence has been obtained, based on robust experimental or observational studies. However, in some areas we have had to rely on expert opinion. Much of the background work was undertaken in the development of evidence-based guidelines for the North Staffordshire project Achieving Sustainable Quality in Maternity (ASQUAM), co-ordinated by Richard Johanson. The Cochrane Database of Systematic Reviews was searched for relevant evidence. A series of MIDIRS Medline searches were used and local Medline searches were undertaken for the remaining topics.

The text covers life-threatening emergencies and where appropriate attention is drawn to their inclusion in the Report on Confidential Enquiries into Maternal Deaths in the United Kingdom 1994–1996. Immediately life-threatening emergencies are grouped together in the 'resuscitation' section. The 'obstetric emergencies' section covers crises peculiar to the obstetric patient. Other emergencies are covered in the 'medical emergencies' section. A small section is included to address matters of medicolegal importance.

The style of topics leads the reader through logical safe steps. It may not be necessary to work through to the end of the plan to restore the patient to a safe condition; this will depend on patient condition and the effectiveness of preceding steps. It is recommended, however, that in a moment of less stress the rest of the chapter is consulted for practical background information.

We make no apology for the repetition from chapter to chapter of basic life-saving drill. Such information is at hand whenever it might be needed.

Drugs which will be changing names in accordance with the Directive 92/27/EEC have been referred to by both their UK name and their Recommended International Non-proprietary Name.

Names of authors are given at the beginning of some chapters. Where no names are given the chapter was written by the main authors.

We would like to thank Claire Rigby (ASQUAM coordinator) for producing the series of ASQUAM guidelines utilized in this book. We would also like to thank Andy Pickersgill and Tim Craft for their comments on the manuscript.

Charles Cox
Kate Grady
Richard Johanson

ACKNOWLEDGEMENTS

We would like to acknowledge the generosity of the following organizations who have given permission for their material to be reproduced in this book.

European Resuscitation Council (Figure 1, page 11)

Bossaert *et al.* (1998) European Resuscitation Council guidelines for the use of automated external defibrillators by EMS providers and first responders. *Resuscitation* **37**: 91–94.

European Resuscitation Council (Figure 2, page 12)

C. Robertson *et al.* (1998) The 1998 European Resuscitation Council guidelines for adult advanced life support. *Resuscitation* **37**: 81–90.

European Resuscitation Council (Figures 1–3, pages 17–19)

D. Chamberlain *et al.* (1994) Peri-arrest arrhythmias (management of arrhythmias associated with cardiac arrest). A statement by the Advanced Life Support Committee of the European Resuscitation Council. *Resuscitation* **28**: 151–159.

D. Chamberlain *et al.* (1996) Peri-arrest arrhythmias: notice of 1st update. *Resuscitation* **31**: 281.

The Association of Anaesthetists of Great Britain and Ireland (pages 133–136)

The 'Anaphylaxis' topic is based on the 1995 publication *Suspected Anaphylactic Reactions Associated with Anaesthesia*.

Birmingham Women's Hospital

The normal values on the inside back cover are taken from an internal publication.

FOREWORD

Thankfully, obstetric emergencies are reasonably uncommon, but when they do occur they are often unexpected and can develop rapidly. Their relative rareness means that midwives and medical attendants may not be sufficiently practised to deal with them efficiently and effectively, and under these circumstances a potentially survivable condition can lead to maternal death or morbidity.

The problem of adequate training and the maintenance of skills amongst attendants can be dealt with in a number of ways. This book provides the framework for the management of a variety of obstetric and medical emergencies. Courses are now run in the UK, one of which is organized in the West Midlands by the contributors to this book, that provide an opportunity to practice some of the basic resuscitation and operative techniques required. Finally, the RCOG document on 'Towards Safer Childbirth' recommends that dummy obstetric emergencies be held regularly – the contents of this book could form a helpful basis for labour ward protocols in this area.

The authors are to be congratulated on producing a practically useful book which reflects the fact that they themselves are active daily at the obstetric 'front line'. It should prove a useful source of guidance and information for midwives and obstetricians.

Professor MJ Whittle

AIRWAY OBSTRUCTION

Airway obstruction must be suspected when **breath sounds are absent or noisy or if the patient is cyanosed**. Airway obstruction is likely to occur in the unconscious patient. If breathing is compromised the patient *may* have an airway problem or it may have a respiratory, cardiovascular, neurological or metabolic cause. Obstruction of the airway results in compromise to oxygenation with consequent maternal and fetal hypoxia. The completely obstructed airway will cause maternal neurological or other vital system damage in 2–5 min.

ACTION PLAN

1 **Shake the patient and shout**
- 'Are you all right?'
- Look for chest movements/muscle activity.
- Listen for breath sounds and other noises.
- Feel for movement of air from the mouth and nose.

Look, listen and feel for up to 10 sec before deciding that breathing is absent.

2 **Call for help including resident anaesthetist**

3 **Open airway**
- Head tilt (omit if suspicion of cervical spine injury).
- Chin lift.
- Jaw thrust.

4 **Reassess**
- Look for chest movements.
- Listen for breath sounds.
- Feel for movement of air.

5 **If breathing and conscious**
- Apply oxygen 15 l/min via tight fitting face mask with reservoir bag.
- Do not disturb position.
- Attach pulse oximeter to patient which should read >93%.
- Further assess.

6 **If breathing and unconscious**
- Apply oxygen.
- Put in recovery position on left side.
- Attach pulse oximeter to patient.
- Further assess.

7 **If not breathing**
- Turn to supine position (slightly tilted to patient's left if another rescuer available and use manual in-line stabilization of the head and neck if a cervical spine injury suspected).
- Remove any visible obstruction from mouth.

8 **Ventilate with face mask and self-inflating bag attached to oxygen flow at 15 l/min** (or mouth to mouth, mouth to nose or

mouth to mask if equipment not immediately available) maintaining head tilt, chin lift and jaw thrust

9 **During ventilation maintain cricoid pressure**

10 **If unable to ventilate**
- Check adequate head tilt, chin lift jaw thrust.
- Place oropharyngeal airway.

11 **If still unable to ventilate, intubate the patient if you are appropriately trained** – *do not use drugs* unless you are an anaesthetist

12 **If unable to intubate try placing laryngeal mask airway, pharyngotracheal lumen airway or oesophageal/tracheal combitube attached to self-inflating bag and oxygen**

13 **If unable to ventilate with these perform cricothyroidotomy**
- This must be followed by tracheal intubation.

14 **Check circulation; CPR if necessary, secure i.v. access, run i.v.i.**

15 **Check CTG – if fetal compromise, immediate delivery should be considered**

16 **Further assess**
- Cause of airway obstruction.

17 **Arrange ICU if intubated, tracheostomy or residual airway problem**

18 **Keep record chart of pulse, BP, RR, SaO$_2$, FH and treatments given**

19 **Document in notes, with time, date, a signature and printed identification and inform consultant obstetrician and consultant anaesthetist**

CONSULT OTHER TOPICS

Amniotic fluid embolism (p. 47)
Anaphylaxis (p. 133)
Cardiopulmonary resuscitation (p. 8)
Eclampsia, pre-eclampsia, HELLP, fatty liver and hepatic rupture (p. 66)
Loss of consciousness or fitting (p. 157)
Respiratory emergencies (p. 20)
Spinals and epidurals – high spinal anaesthesia (p. 169)
Spinals and epidurals – local anaesthetic toxicity (p. 171)
Thromboembolism (p. 177)

SUPPLEMENTARY INFORMATION

Assess airway

If the patient is able to respond verbally, if there are chest movements, breath sounds and the movement of air is felt at the nose and mouth, the airway is not completely obstructed. It may be partially obstructed however. Indrawing of the abdominal wall, the intercostal and tracheal areas, absent or noisy breath sounds are signs of partial airway obstruction.

Open airway

Head tilt

Place hand on forehead and gently tilt head back.

Chin lift

At the same time as the head tilt place fingertips under the point of patient's chin and lift chin forward. The thumb of the same hand lightly depresses the jaw to open the mouth.

Jaw thrust

Grasp the angles of the lower jaw, one hand each side and pull the jaw forwards, lightly depressing the lower lip.

If breathing and unconscious

- Apply oxygen.
- Put in recovery position on left side.

Recovery position

- Remove spectacles.
- Kneel on the left side of patient and make sure both her legs are straight.
- Open airway.
- Tuck patient's left hand, arm straight and palm uppermost, well under patient's buttock.
- Bring the right arm across the chest and hold the back of the hand against the patient's left cheek.
- With your other hand grasp the right leg just above the knee and pull it up, keeping the foot on the ground.
- Keeping the patient's hand pressed against the cheek, pull on the right leg to roll the patient onto her left side.
- Adjust right leg so hip and knee are bent at right angles.
- Adjust the left arm so patient not lying on it and palm still uppermost.
- Ensure head tilt, chin lift and jaw thrust, using the hand under the cheek if necessary to keep head tilted.
- Check breathing.

If not breathing

Turn to supine position and remove any visible obstruction from mouth.

- Gently clear secretions with suction.
- If foreign body and air movement encourage the patient to cough and apply oxygen via tight fitting mask and reservoir bag at a flow of 15 l/min and further assess.
- If foreign body and movement of air is poor or absent or the patient is cyanosed, try to clear the obstruction by head and neck alignment, back blows, chest thrusts, finger sweeps of the mouth, using a laryngoscope with suction or forceps to remove the obstruction. May need to proceed to cricothyroidotomy.

To carry out back blows stand to the side and slightly behind patient. Support the chest with one hand and lean the patient forwards. Give up to five sharp blows between the scapulae with the heel of the other hand. If back blows fail, carry out chest thrusts by applying rhythmic thrusts with both hands to the anterior aspect of the chest in the same position used for external chest compressions. Finger sweeps should only be used in the unconscious patient.

Ventilate with face mask and self-inflating bag attached to oxygen at a flow of 15 l/min

If you are able to, ventilate the patient by face mask and self-inflating bag; tracheal intubation, however, remains the optimal procedure: summon an anaesthetist to do this. Ventilation must be continued until this is accomplished. A patient with obtunded laryngeal or pharyngeal reflexes (unconscious or hypotensive) is at risk of aspiration of regurgitated fluids. Their airway may be patent or may require support but they also require protection of the airway and therefore intubation is always necessary.

During ventilation maintain cricoid pressure

Cricoid pressure is used to prevent aspiration of regurgitated gastric contents. It should not compromise ventilation which is the primary goal.

If unable to ventilate, check adequate head tilt, chin lift, jaw thrust, and place oropharyngeal airway

Oropharyngeal airways can only be used in unconscious patients.

If unable to intubate try placing laryngeal mask airway, pharyngotracheal lumen airway or oesophogeal/tracheal combitube attached to self-inflating bag and oxygen

The laryngeal mask is the method of choice; the others require more training.

If unable to ventilate with these perform cricothyroidotomy

This should not be undertaken lightly. It is indicated when it is impossible to make the airway patent by other methods.

If an emergency cricothyroidotomy kit is not available, an intravenous cannula is inserted through the cricothyroid membrane. The cricothyroid membrane lies between the thyroid cartilage (Adam's apple) and the cricoid cartilage (the cartilage immediately inferior to the Adam's apple). This can be attached to oxygen tubing with a hole cut towards one end attached to the wall source of oxygen. Intermittent ventilation can be achieved by occluding the hole for 1 sec and releasing it for 4 sec. This technique buys time only until tracheal intubation. Care should be taken in complete airway obstruction to avoid a build up of pressure within the chest.

Tracheostomy should only be performed by a suitably skilled person.

Check CTG – if fetal compromise, immediate delivery should be considered

The priority is to adequately oxygenate the mother. Do not deliver the baby if this presents further compromise to maternal oxygenation.

If the mother is being adequately oxygenated but the airway is unprotected, i.e. she does not have a cuffed tube in her trachea, it is reasonable to proceed to delivery. This should not delay providing the mother with a protected airway (cuffed tube in trachea).

Causes of airway obstruction:

- Tongue displacement as in the unconscious or hypotensive.
- Soft tissue oedema as in anaphylaxis.
- Soft tissue swelling or displacement as in trauma.
- Foreign body.

REFERENCES

Baskett PJF, Bossaert L, Carli P *et al.* (1996) Guidelines for the advanced management of the airway and ventilation during resuscitation. A statement by the Airway and Ventilation Mangement Group of the European Resuscitation Council. *Resuscitation* **31**: 201–230.

Committee on Trauma (1997) *Advanced Trauma Life Support for Doctors*. American College of Surgeons.

European Resuscitation Council (1998) *Guidelines for adult advanced life support. Resuscitation* **37**: 81–90.

Gabbott DA and PJF Baskett (1997) Management of the airway and ventilation during resuscitation. *Br. J. Anaesth.* **79**: 159–171.

Nolan JR and Parr MJA (1997) Aspects of resuscitation in trauma. *Br. J. Anaesth.* **79**: 226–240.

Resuscitation Council (1997) *The 1997 Resuscitation Guidelines for use in the United Kingdom.*

BURNS

ACTION PLAN

1 Assess and ensure patency of airway (cervical spine control)

2 Consider early intubation if burns to airway or smoke inhalation

3 Administer oxygen 15 l/min via tight fitting face mask with reservoir bag

4 Check arterial blood gases for carboxyhaemoglobin levels

5 Assess and assist breathing

6 Assess circulatory status and evaporative losses

7 Consider presence of other injuries and treat

8 Assess need to deliver the fetus

9 Remove all clothes and keep warm

10 Consider need for escharotomies

11 Cover burns with clean dressings

12 Keep a record chart to include pulse, BP, RR, SaO_2, FH, urine output, carboxyhaemoglobin levels, exhaled CO_2 and treatments given

13 Document degree and extent of burn and treatment concisely and chronologically in notes with time, date, a signature and printed identification and inform consultant obstetrician

14 Transfer to another centre if necessary

CONSULT OTHER TOPICS

Eclampsia, pre-eclampsia, HELLP, fatty liver and hepatic rupture (p. 66)
Loss of consciousness or fitting (p. 157)
Neonatal resuscitation (p. 14)
Puerperal sepsis, septicaemia and septic shock (p. 113)

SUPPLEMENTARY INFORMATION

Check arterial blood gases for carboxyhaemoglobin levels

If an inhalational injury is suspected. Note the time of the burn and the time the arterial sample was taken.

Assess circulatory status and evaporative losses

- By heart rate, urine output, BP and 'rule of nines'. Place urinary catheter to monitor output – aim for 50 ml/hour.
- Secure i.v. access and replace fluids with warmed crystalloid solution.
- Replace fluid. The patient requires 2–4 ml/kg/per cent of body surface area burned in the first 24 hours after the burn. Half of this volume is given in the first 8 hours following the burn and half in the next 16 hours. The body surface area burned is estimated by the 'rule of nines'. Parts of the body are divided into areas of 9% (or multiples of 9%) of total surface area. For example, back is 18%, leg is 18%, arm is 9% (palm is 1%).

Assess need to deliver the fetus

- Pregnancy does not affect maternal outcome of burns.
- The fetal prognosis relates to the extent of the burn.
- The prognosis for the fetus depends on maternal complications such as hypoxia, hypotension and sepsis.
- Abortion is common in patients with burns exceeding 33% of body surface area, especially during the second trimester.
- Fetal loss during the third trimester can be expected with burns exceeding 33% of body surface unless delivery occurs within 5 days.

ELECTRICAL BURNS

- There is limited data.
- The amniotic fluid and uterus are good conductors of electricity.
- There are reports of long-term oligohydramnios and intrauterine growth retardation, but it is generally felt that there is an all or nothing effect on the fetus – either death results or the prognosis is comparatively good.

Consider need for escharotomies

Burned tissue may constrict the blood supply to the limbs. The procedure of cutting through burned tissue to restore blood supply is called escharotomy. Call for general surgical assistance.

REFERENCES

Committee on Trauma (1997) *Advanced Trauma Life Support for Doctors*. American College of Surgeons.

CARDIOPULMONARY RESUSCITATION

The patient appears lifeless. There is loss of consciousness, no breathing and no circulation.

1   **Ensure safe environment for victim and rescuer(s)**

2   **Shout and shake 'Are you all right?'**

3   **If patient responds**
   - Place in left lateral position.
   - Send for help if necessary.
   - Assess breathing, pulse, BP and FH.
   - Regularly reassess.

4   **If no response, get help. If alone, call help before attending to patient**

5   **Open airway by head tilt, chin lift and assess breathing for 10 seconds**
   - Look for chest movements.
   - Listen for breath sounds.
   - Feel for the movement of air.

6   **If breathing**
   - Place in left lateral position.
   - Ensure help on the way if necessary.
   - Assess breathing, pulse, BP and FH.
   - Regularly reassess.

7   **If automatic external defibrillator (AED) available, attach, analyse rhythm and defibrillate if indicated (see *Figure 1* p. 11)**

8   **If not breathing**
   - Ensure help is on its way.
   - Turn patient onto back.
   - Open airway.
   - Remove any obstruction from patient's mouth.

9   **Give two rescue breaths**
   - Make no more than five attempts to achieve two breaths; if unsuccessful move on to 10.

10 **Assess for signs of circulation for *no more* than 10 seconds**
   - Look for any movement including swallowing or breathing.
   - Check the carotid pulse.

11 **If circulation present but no breathing continue rescue breathing at a rate of 10 breaths/min**
   - Recheck the presence of circulation every 10 breaths.

12 **If no circulation start chest compressions after two initial breaths**
- Perform 15 chest compressions.
- Continue this cycle of two breaths to 15 chest compressions.
- With two rescuers alter the cycle to one breath to five chest compressions.
- Compressions should be about 100/min.

13 **Continue until signs of life or help arrives to provide advanced life support**

14 **Ensure cardiac arrest team on their way. Call for senior obstetrician and obstetric anaesthetist**

15 **Ensure wedge or manual displacement of uterus to the left**

16 **Attach defibrillator/monitor and assess cardiac rhythm**

17 **Turn immediately to advanced life support (ALS) algorithm (*Figure 2*, p. 12)**
- Each step that follows in the ALS algorithm assumes that the preceding one has been unsuccessful.
- Adrenaline/epinephrine 1 mg i.v. should be given at the completion of each loop.
- Chest compressions may be less effective in the presence of spinal or epidural block – larger doses of adrenaline/epinephrine may be necessary therefore.
- Cardiovascular collapse due to bupivacaine toxicity requires prolonged resuscitation and the use of bretylium.

18 **Consider and treat cause of cardiac arrest**

19 **Perform emergency Caesarean section** (if aggressive CPR with properly positioned patient not successful after 5 min)

20 **Make decision to abandon CPR if unsuccessful** (resuscitation should continue for 20–30 min from the time of collapse, unless there are overwhelming reasons to believe it to be futile)

21 **Keep record chart of events and treatments**

22 **Record in notes and report to consultant obstetrician if not present. Inform coroner if necessary**

CONSULT OTHER TOPICS

Airway obstruction (p. 1)
Eclampsia, pre-eclampsia, HELLP, fatty liver and hepatic rupture (p. 66)
Hypotension (p. 150)
Massive obstetric haemorrhage – DIC (p. 92)
Peri-arrest arrhythmias (p. 16)
Thromboembolism (p. 177)
Spinals and epidurals – high spinal anaesthesia (p. 169)
Spinals and epidurals – local anaesthetic toxicity (p. 171)
Trauma (p. 24)

SUPPLEMENTARY INFORMATION

Points 1–12 follow the Basic Life Support Guidelines of the European Resuscitation Council 1998.

Point 15 follows the Advanced Life Support Guidelines.

If patient responds

- Place in the left lateral position to avoid supine hypotension.
- Apply oxygen at 15 l/min by face mask with reservoir bag.

Open airway by head tilt, chin lift and assess breathing for 10 sec

- Do this with the patient in the position in which you find her.
- Do this (but not if cervical spine injury is suspected), by placing hand on the forehead and gently tilting head back keeping thumb and index finger free to close the patient's nose if rescue breathing is required. At the same time with your fingertips under the point of the patient's chin, lift the chin to open the airway. A jaw thrust may be required to open the airway. Do this by placing fingers behind the angle of the jaws and moving jaw anteriorly to displace tongue from the pharynx.
- If you have any difficulty, turn the patient onto her back with a slight tilt to the left and then open the airway as described. Try to avoid head tilt if injury to the neck is suspected.

If automatic external defibrillator (AED) available, attach, analyse rhythm and defibrillate if indicated

The most frequent initial rhythm in cardiac arrest is ventricular fibrillation (VF). Successful defibrillation diminishes with time. The AED allows for early defibrillation by lesser trained personnel as it performs rhythm analysis, gives information by voice or visual display and the delivery of the shock is then delivered manually. After the first three shocks give uninterrupted CPR for 1 min. If defibrillation is not indicated CPR should be continued for 3 min at which stage the AED will prompt further analysis of rhythm.

Give two rescue breaths

Do this by ensuring head tilt and chin lift, and closing the soft part of the patient's nose with your thumb and index finger, with the palm of your hand on the patient's forehead. Open her mouth a little but maintain chin lift. Take a breath and place your lips around her mouth, making sure that you have a good seal. Blow steadily into her mouth over 1.5–2 sec, watching for her chest to rise. The target tidal volume is 400–500 ml. Maintaining head tilt and chin lift, take your mouth away from the patient and watch for her chest to fall as the air comes out. Take another breath and repeat the sequence to give another effective breath. If you have difficulty in achieving a breath, recheck the patient's mouth for an obstruction, and ensure that head tilt and chin lift are adequate.

If circulation present but no breathing continue rescue breathing at a rate of 10 breaths/min

Recheck the circulation every 10 breaths, taking no more than 10 sec each time. If the patient starts to breath on her own but remains unconscious turn her into the recovery position and apply oxygen 15 l/min. Check her condition and be ready to turn her back to restart rescue breathing if she stops breathing.

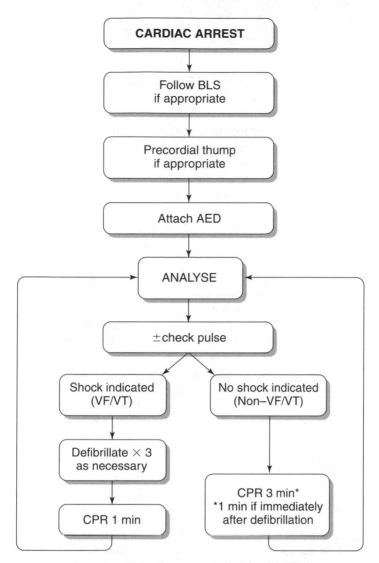

Continue AED algorithm until ALS available

Figure 1. Automatic external defibrillator (AED) algorithm.

If no circulation (or you are at all unsure) start chest compressions after two initial breaths

With the patient tilted to the left, locate the lower half of the sternum: using your index and middle fingers identify the lower rib margins. Keeping your fingers together slide them up to the point where the ribs join the sternum. With your middle finger on this point place your index finger on the sternum.

Slide the heel of your other hand down the sternum until it reaches your index finger; this should be the middle of the lower half of the sternum.

Place the heel of one hand there, with the other hand on top of the first.

Interlock the fingers of both hands and lift them to ensure that pressure is not applied over the patient's ribs. Do not apply any pressure over the top of the abdomen or bottom tip of the sternum.

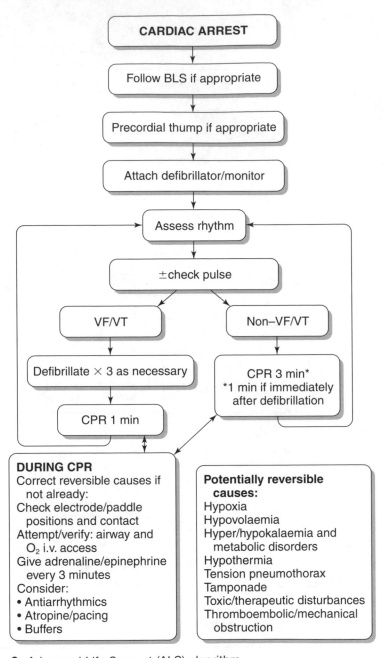

Figure 2. Advanced Life Support (ALS) algorithm.

Position yourself above the patient's chest and with your arms straight press down on the sternum to depress it 4–5 cm.

Release the pressure then repeat at a rate of about 100 times a minute. Compression and release should take an equal amount of time.

To combine rescue breathing and compression after 15 compressions tilt the head, lift the chin and give two effective breaths. Return your hands immediately to the correct position and give 15 further compressions continuing this cycle of two breaths to 15 compressions.

Two person CPR is preferred if there are two rescuers. A ratio of five compressions to one ventilation should be used.

Attach defibrillator/monitor and assess cardiac rhythm

For defibrillation one paddle is placed to the right of the upper part of the sternum just below the clavicle, the other just outside the position of the normal cardiac apex, taking care to avoid breast tissue.

Turn immediately to advanced life support (ALS) algorithm (p. 12)

The majority of patients will have been successfully defibrillated in one of the first three defibrillating shocks. If the patient remains in VF a successful outcome relies on continued defibrillation and correction of causes or contributing factors. Antiarrhythmic agents should be prescribed by the medical registrar only. Sodium bicarbonate should only be given to patients with severe acidosis pH < 7.1; base excess < −10.

If VF/VT can be positively excluded, defibrillation is not indicated. The patient is in asystole or electromechanical dissociation (EMD). The causes of cardiac arrest are hypovolaemia, total spinal anaesthetic or local anaesthetic toxicity, pneumothorax, cardiac tamponade, massive pulmonary embolus or amniotic fluid embolus, or eclampsia.

Perform emergency Caesarean section

This will reduce maternal oxygen consumption, increase venous return, make ventilation easier and allow for CPR in the supine position. A vertical abdominal and uterine incision should be used for speed. Consider open cardiac massage .

Make decision to abandon CPR if unsuccessful

Do not abandon CPR if rhythm continues as VF/VT. Decision to abandon CPR should only be made after discussion with consultant obstetrician and senior clinicians.

REFERENCES

Advanced Life Support Working Group of the European Resuscitation Council (1998) The 1998 European Resuscitation Council guidelines for adult advanced life support. *Br. Med. J.* **316**: 1863–1870.

Basic Life Support Working Group of the European Resuscitation Council (1998) The 1998 European Resuscitation Council guidelines for adult single rescuer basic life support. *Br. Med. J.* **316**: 1870–1876.

Robertson C *et al.* (1998) The 1998 European Resuscitation Council guidelines for adult advanced life support. *Resuscitation* **37 (2)**: 81–90.

NEONATAL RESUSCITATION

E. O'Donnell

It is important where possible to predict the need for basic or advanced life support for the neonate. Good communication is essential between those involved in the care of the mother and those to be involved in the care of the baby. Obstetricians should discuss the maternal and fetal condition with paediatricians prenatally to allow time to prepare for the problems which may arise. This also ensures that time is available for the paediatricians to have a detailed discussion with the family.

ACTION PLAN

1 **Prepare for resuscitation – call paediatrician urgently**

2 **At birth determine the Apgar score and note the time**

3 **Dry neonate and wrap in warm towel**

4 **If meconium present consider suction of trachea before stimulation**

5 **If baby does not cry stimulate gently by more vigorous drying or flicking the soles of the feet**

6 **If gasping or not breathing follow ABCs**

7 **Open airway by head tilt, chin lift or jaw thrust**

8 **Suction carefully**

9 **Consider naloxone**

10 **If still not breathing ventilate with bag–valve–mask at 30–60 breaths/min**

11 **If still not breathing intubate the trachea and ventilate**

12 **If heart rate is < 60 beats/min start chest compressions 100/min**

13 **If heart rate fails to respond to effective ventilation and chest compressions cannulate the umbilical cord and consider adrenaline/epinephrine 0.1 ml/kg of a 1:10 000 solution**

14 **Consider expansion of circulating volume with 10 ml/kg of cross-matched blood or albumin**

15 **Document resuscitation concisely and chronologically in notes with date, a signature and printed identification**

SUPPLEMENTARY INFORMATION

Prepare for resuscitation

- Anticipate problems.
- Call for help.

- Check equipment – ensure that the radiant heater is on, the oxygen supply is connected and working, the pressure valve is set at 30 cm of water, the laryngoscope is working, the suction is functioning, endotrachial tubes are available, and that emergency drugs are available.

At birth determine the Apgar score and note the time

Apgar scores at 20 min are more strongly predictive of poor outcome than earlier scores. Change in score over time may be useful in providing a guide to the success of resuscitation.

Apgar scoring system

Score	Pulse	Respiratory effort	Muscle tone	Colour	Reflex irritability
2	>100	Strong cry	Active movement	Pink	Cry
1	<100	Irregular	Limb flexion	Body pink	Grimace
0	Absent	Nil	Absent	Blue	Nil

If meconium present consider suction of trachea before stimulation

During oropharyngeal suction the catheter should not go further than 5 cm.

Deeper prolonged suction may cause laryngospasm, bradycardia, and even cardiac arrhythmia due to vagal stimulation.

If there is meconium, aspirate the pharynx as the head is delivered. Meconium aspiration should be assessed by direct laryngoscopy. If there is evidence of meconium in the trachea, elective intubation and direct suctioning of the trachea is required.

If still not breathing ventilate with bag–valve–mask at 30–60 breaths/min

Ensure the system has a reservoir bag and a blow off valve set to 30 cm of water to minimize the risk of pneumothorax. The mask should cover the mouth and nose but not the chin or eyes.

When the heart rate is above 100 beats/min and the infant becomes pink and makes spontaneous respiratory effort, bagging should be discontinued and oxygen alone given.

If still not breathing intubate the trachea and ventilate

Infants who remain apnoeic, those with Apgar scores less than 3, and those who can not maintain a heart rate above 100 beats/min with assisted ventilation using a bag and mask will require intubation (if someone with this skill is at hand).

Use a 3.5 mm tube on term infants. For birth weights 1250–2500 g use 3.0 mm. A size 2.5 may be used on infants with a weight less than 1250 g.

If heart rate is < 60 beats/min start chest compressions

Cardiac massage is performed by encircling the infants body with both hands, with the thumbs at the mid-sternal notch (nipple line). The chest is compressed at a rate of 100–120 beats/min. Give three chest compressions for each ventilation.

REFERENCE

Zideman D A (1997) Paediatric and neonatal life support. *Br. J. Anaesth.* **79**: 178–187.

Neonatal Resuscitation

PERI-ARREST ARRHYTHMIAS

S. Maguire and K. Grady

A peri-arrest arrhythmia refers to a malignant cardiac rhythm which may lead to cardiac arrest or a rhythm which occurs following resuscitation from cardiac arrest.

Normally

1 A P wave precedes each QRS complex and is upright in leads lll and AVF.
2 The PR interval is 0.12–0.2 sec (3–5 small squares).
3 The QRS complex is less than 0.08 sec (2 small squares).

The standard speed for recording an ECG is 25 mm/sec. At this rate one large square represents 0.2 sec and one small square represents 0.04 sec.

Arrhythmias are broadly categorized into

- Bradycardia, which is usually defined as a heart rate of less than 60 beats/ minute. In the term pregnant patient the heart rate is increased by approximately 15% so a rate greater than 60 beats/minute may represent a relative bradycardia. In the presence of hypotension, consider that a heart rate greater than 60 beats/minute may be inappropriately slow and may require treatment.
- Two types of tachyarrhythmias, conventionally divided into those that arise within the ventricle (ventricular tachycardias) or above (supraventricular tachycardias). Accurate classification of the origin of the tachycardia may be difficult. The following guidelines therefore make no assumption that the origin of the tachycardia has been defined accurately. Treatment is based on the simple classification of narrow QRS complex tachycardias (usually supraventricular and may be treated as such with acceptable safety) and broad QRS complex tachycardias (which are assumed to be ventricular).

<table>
<tr><td rowspan="5">ACTION PLAN</td><td>1</td><td>Call for help including cardiac arrest team, senior obstetrician and obstetric anaesthetist</td></tr>
<tr><td>2</td><td>If bradycardia, follow the algorithm on p. 17 (Figure 1). If not already done, give oxygen and establish i.v. access. Doses are based on an adult of average bodyweight

If broad complex tachycardia (sustained ventricular tachycardia), follow the algorithm on p. 18 (Figure 2). If not already done, give oxygen and establish i.v. access. Doses are based on an adult of average bodyweight

If narrow complex tachycardia (supraventricular tachycardia), follow the algorithm on p. 19 (Figure 3). If not already done, give oxygen and establish i.v. access. Doses are based on an adult of average bodyweight</td></tr>
<tr><td>3</td><td>Continuously monitor fetal heart by cardiotocography and consider timing and method of delivery</td></tr>
<tr><td>4</td><td>Keep a record of sequence of above drills and FH</td></tr>
<tr><td>5</td><td>Document in notes with times, date, a signature and printed identification and report to consultant obstetrician</td></tr>
</table>

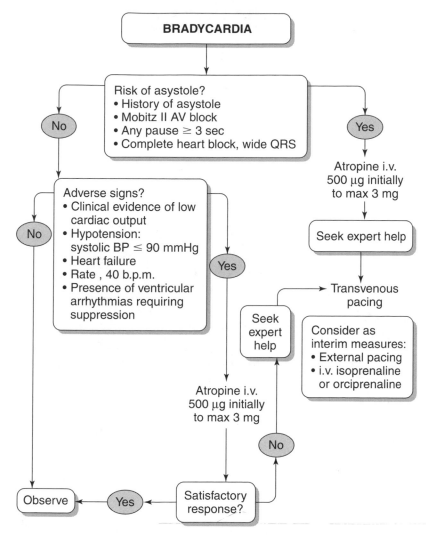

Figure 1. Algorithm for bradycardia.

CONSULT OTHER TOPICS

Airway obstruction (p. 1)
Cardiopulmonary resuscitation (p. 8)
Hypotension (p. 150)
Respiratory emergencies (p. 20)

SUPPLEMENTARY INFORMATION

All antiarrhythmic strategies can be proarrhythmic. Deterioration can occur as a result of treatment and treatment can cause myocardial depression and hypotension. How far sequential treatments should be pursued in the face of these risks is a matter of clinical judgment.

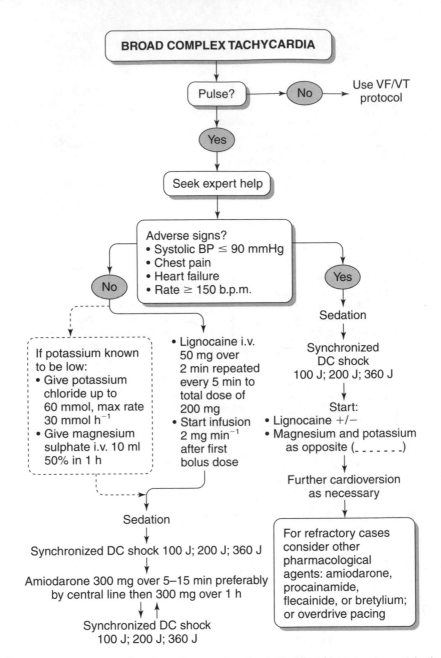

Figure 2. Algorithm for broad complex tachycardia (sustained ventricular tachycardia).

REFERENCE

Advanced Life Support Working Party of the European Resuscitation Council (1994) Peri-arrest arrhythmias: notice of 1st update. *Resuscitation* **31**: 281.

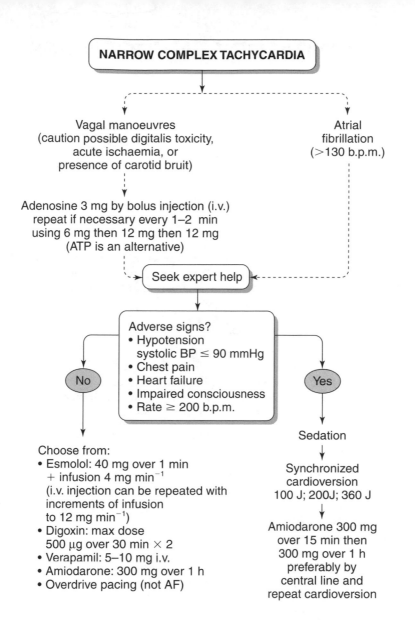

NARROW COMPLEX TACHYCARDIA

Vagal manoeuvres
(caution possible digitalis toxicity,
acute ischaemia, or
presence of carotid bruit)

Atrial
fibrillation
(>130 b.p.m.)

Adenosine 3 mg by bolus injection (i.v.)
repeat if necessary every 1–2 min
using 6 mg then 12 mg then 12 mg
(ATP is an alternative)

Seek expert help

Adverse signs?
• Hypotension
  systolic BP ≤ 90 mmHg
• Chest pain
• Heart failure
• Impaired consciousness
• Rate ≥ 200 b.p.m.

No

Yes

Choose from:
• Esmolol: 40 mg over 1 min
  + infusion 4 mg min^{-1}
  (i.v. injection can be repeated with
  increments of infusion
  to 12 mg min^{-1})
• Digoxin: max dose
  500 µg over 30 min × 2
• Verapamil: 5–10 mg i.v.
• Amiodarone: 300 mg over 1 h
• Overdrive pacing (not AF)

Sedation

Synchronized
cardioversion
100 J; 200J; 360 J

Amiodarone 300 mg
over 15 min then
300 mg over 1 h
preferably by
central line and
repeat cardioversion

Notes: *Vagal manoeuvres include the Valsalva manoeuvre, and
carotid sinus massage (performed unilaterally and only
after a carotid bruit has been excluded).
β-blockade after verapamil may result in AV node standstill.*

Figure 3. Algorithm for narrow complex tachycardia (supraventricular tachycardia).

RESPIRATORY EMERGENCIES

Signs of respiratory insufficiency are

- absent breath sounds
- noisy breathing (stridor or wheeze)
- breathlessness
- shallow breathing
- slow respiratory rate (< 8 breaths/min)
- cyanosis
- tachycardia

These signs may also be due to airway compromise. Airway compromise will kill or damage the patient more quickly than a respiratory problem. An airway problem must therefore be excluded or attended to at the outset.

1 **Exclude an airway problem**

2 **Assess breathing**
- 'Are you all right?'
- Look for chest movements, pink frothy sputum.
- Listen for breath sounds or noises associated with breathing.
- Feel for the movement of air from the mouth and nose.

Look, listen and feel for up to 10 sec before deciding that breathing is absent.

3 **Call for help including resident anaesthetist**

4 **If breathing and conscious**
- Apply oxygen 15 l/min via tight fitting face mask with reservoir bag.
- Sit upright.
- Attach pulse oximeter to patient which should read >94%, NIBP and ECG monitor.
- Further assess with anaesthetist; consider need for continuous positive airways pressure (CPAP) or intubation.
- If breathing patient becomes apnoeic, ventilate and intubate.
- Consider cause of respiratory distress.

5 **If breathing and unconscious**
- Apply oxygen 15 l/min via tight fitting face mask with reservoir bag.
- Put in recovery position on left side.
- Attach pulse oximeter which should read >94%, NIBP and ECG monitor.
- Call anaesthetist to intubate.
- Further assess.
- If breathing patient becomes apnoeic, ventilate and intubate.
- Consider cause of respiratory distress.

6 **If not breathing**
- Turn to supine position (slightly tilted to patient's left if another

rescuer available and use manual in-line stabilization of the head and neck if a cervical spine injury suspected).

- Open airway.

7 **Ventilate with face mask and self-inflating bag attached to oxygen flow at 15 l/min** (or mouth to mouth, mouth to nose or mouth to mask if equipment not immediately available), maintaining head tilt, chin lift and jaw thrust

8 **During ventilation maintain cricoid pressure**

9 **Check circulation**, CPR if necessary, secure i.v. access, send bloods for FBC, U&Es, cardiac enzymes and blood glucose, run i.v.i. slowly

10 **Arrange urgent tracheal intubation** to provide the means of ventilation *and* to protect the airway as she is unconscious. Ventilation must be continued until this is achieved

11 **Endotracheal intubation** – *do not use drugs* unless you are an anaesthetist

12 **Request ABGs, CXR and ECG**

13 **Call physician and treat underlying condition**

14 **Check fetal heart and continuously monitor by cardiotocography. Consider timing and method of delivery**

15 **Arrange ICU** if intubated or residual respiratory compromise

16 **Keep a record chart to include pulse, RR, SaO$_2$, BP, FH and treatments given**

17 **Document in notes, with time, date, a signature and printed identification and report to consultant obstetrician and consultant anaesthetist**

CONSULT OTHER TOPICS

Respiratory Emergencies

SUPPLEMENTARY INFORMATION

If breathing and conscious/unconscious

Attach pulse oximeter to patient

In all patients aim to keep oxygen saturation >94%. When lower than this there is significant hypoxia and intubation may be required. A decision to intubate a breathing patient should only be taken by an anaesthetist who will give consideration to degree of hypoxia, respiratory reserve and exhaustion.

Consider cause of respiratory distress

Respirations may be slow or shallow or the patient may be struggling for breath.
   Consider whether patient is hypoventilating (slow or shallow breathing).
   Hypoventilation may be due to opioid drugs (i.m., i.v., epidural or spinal) – turn off epidural infusion and give naloxone 100–500 µg i.v. in increments if there is a central nervous system cause.
   If patient is struggling for breath consider following causes

* pulmonary oedema
* pneumothorax
* aspiration pneumonitis
* pulmonary embolus also amniotic fluid embolus, venous air embolus
* pneumonia
* pulmonary contusion
* asthma
* adult respiratory distress syndrome (ARDS)
* anaphylaxis/allergic reaction
* airway obstruction

Pulmonary oedema

This is caused by the transudation of fluid from the alveolar capillaries to the alveolar spaces. This fluid causes a barrier to oxygenation. Pulmonary oedema can occur in pre-eclampsia, septicaemia, following respiratory obstruction, or in left ventricular failure due to peripartum cardiomyopathy, myocardial infarction, pulmonary embolus, fluid overload or valvular disease.
   The patient is clammy, breathless, tachycardic, may have frothy pink sputum at the mouth, prefers to sit upright, has basal crepitations and a triple rhythm.
   CXR shows engorged upper lobe veins, cardiomegaly, Kerley B lines and bilateral pleural effusions.

* Treat as above.
* Summon anaesthetist and physician urgently.
* Consider frusemide/furosemide 40 mg i.v. (repeat as necessary) if BP stable.
* Consider glyceryl trinitrate tablet 300 µg sublingually if BP stable – physician may recommend infusion.
* Consider morphine sulphate 5 mg i.v.
* Identify and treat arrhythmia and give digoxin as indicated 0.5–1.0 mg i.v. in 0.2 mg increments followed by increments of 0.25 mg 4–6 hourly.
* Cardiovert if clinically indicated.

Pneumothorax

A tension pneumothorax is life-threatening. It causes both respiratory and cardiovascular compromise. Its chest signs are deviation of the trachea away from the affected side, reduced expansion on the affected side, hyperresonant percussion note on the affected side and reduced breath sounds on the affected side. Do not wait for CXR to confirm the diagnosis. Decompress immediately by inserting an intravenous cannula through the second intercostal space in the mid-clavicular line on the affected side. This must be followed by placement of a chest drain.

Aspiration pneumonitis

This is caused by the aspiration of gastric contents. The risk is increased by conditions which reduce the level of consciousness of the mother and by general anaesthesia.

It should be suspected where there is respiratory distress of unknown cause and confirmed by ABGs and CXR.

- Treat as above.
- Place patient on left side, head down.
- Suction upper airways.
- Intubate with cuffed tracheal tube (this may require the use of drugs by an anaesthetist).
- Suction down tracheal tube.
- Ventilate with 100% oxygen and positive end expiratory pressure.
- Attach pulse oximeter and check ABGs.
- Get CXR.
- Place nasogastric tube to empty stomach contents.
- Bronchoscopy, pulmonary toilet and physiotherapy as necessary.
- Give sodium citrate, ranitidine and cisapride.
- Treat bronchospasm as indicated.

TRAUMA

In the UK 4–7% of maternal deaths are attributable to trauma. The incidence of domestic violence increases in pregnancy. Maternal physiology protects the mother at the expense of the fetus. The best method of protecting the fetus is to adequately resuscitate the mother. Apparently trivial injuries to the maternal abdomen may result in fetal loss.

ACTION PLAN

1 **Call trauma team**
- Consult senior obstetrician, paediatrician and general surgeon early.

2 **Take history and note mechanism of injury**

3 **Perform primary survey, resuscitate and reevaluate simultaneously**
- A Airway with cervical spine protection.
  Left lateral tilt or displacement of uterus with spine immobilization
- B Breathing and ventilation.
- C Circulation with aggressive volume replacement and haemorrhage control.
- D Disability – neurological assessment.
- E Exposure/environmental control.
- Attach pulse oximeter to patient, non-invasive BP and ECG and cardiotocograph monitor, and monitor exhaled CO_2 if appropriate.
- Consider need for X-rays of lateral cervical spine and anterior-posterior views of chest and pelvis.
- Place gastric tube (oral if suspected base of skull fracture) and urinary catheter and monitor hourly urine output.

4 **Assess fetal well-being and viability**
- Adequately resuscitate mother.
- Use ultrasound to make early assessment of uterine and other abdominal injuries.
- Once fetal heart has been detected institute continuous monitoring by cardiotocograph.
- Make decision whether to interrupt the pregnancy either for fetal or maternal reasons.
- Assess and treat wounds to maternal abdomen.
- Assess fetomaternal haemorrhage.

5 **Perform secondary survey and treat**

6 **When patient status optimized transfer if appropriate**

7 **Keep a record chart to include pulse, BP, RR, SaO$_2$, FH, urine output, exhaled CO_2 and treatments given**

8 **Document injuries, findings and treatment concisely and chronologically in notes with time, date, a signature and printed identification and inform consultant obstetrician**

CONSULT OTHER TOPICS

Acute abdominal pain (p. 44)
Acute chest pain (p. 8)
Airway obstruction (p. 1)
Anaphylaxis (p. 133)
Cardiopulmonary resuscitation (p. 8)
Eclampsia, pre-eclampsia, HELLP, fatty liver and hepatic rupture (p. 66)
Hypotension (p. 150)
Jehovah's Witness patient (p. 153)
Loss of consciousness or fitting (p. 157)
Massive obstetric haemorrhage – DIC (p. 92)
Neonatal resuscitation (p. 14)
Premature labour (p. 110)
Puerperal sepsis, septicaemia and septic shock (p. 113)
Respiratory emergencies (p. 20)

SUPPLEMENTARY INFORMATION

Take history and note mechanism of injury

- Mechanism, injuries, symptoms and signs, treatment (MIST).
- Consider pre-injury condition.
- Note mechanism of injury ('read the wreckage') e.g. deceleration injury, direct impact, penetrating injury, stab wound, bullet or projectile, domestic violence.

Perform primary survey, resuscitate and reevaluate simultaneously

Adopt ABCDE approach to evaluation and treatment to ensure the greatest threat to life is treated first.

A *Airway with cervical spine protection*

Assess airway
　'Are you all right?'
　look
　listen
　feel

Open airway
　take care not to cause movement of the cervical spine
　chin lift
　jaw thrust
　suction
　oropharyngeal airway
　nasopharyngeal airway
　tracheal intubation
　cricothyroidotomy if necessary

Supplemental oxygen is *always* required via tight fitting face mask and reservoir bag at a flow of 15 l/min.

Protect airway if the patient is unconscious, by tracheal intubation using a cuffed tube and hyperventilate to minimize the brain injury.

If an injury to the cervical spine is suspected (pain in neck, high velocity injury, blunt injury above the clavicle, altered level of consciousness, multiple injuries) the cervical spine must be protected by either

- manual in-line immobilization of the neck,
- or the placement of a hard cervical spine collar, two sand bags on either side of the head and tape across the forehead to attach the head to the sand bags.

Left lateral tilt or displacement of uterus with spine immobilization

Uterine compression of the inferior vena cava can significantly reduce venous return and thereby reduce cardiac output. To prevent this, unless a spinal injury is suspected the pregnant patient should be positioned on her left side. If a spinal injury is suspected, she should be positioned supine, the right hip elevated by 4–6 inches by a towel and the uterus displaced manually to the left side.

B   Breathing and ventilation

Adequate oxygenation can only be achieved with a patent airway and adequate ventilation.

Ensure the airway is patent and assess ventilation as follows

- look for chest movements
- listen for breath sounds
- feel for movement of air from the mouth and nose
- look for obvious chest injuries and for movement of the chest
- feel for equality of chest expansion and surgical emphysema
- percuss to exclude air or blood in the chest
- auscultate

Assist ventilation if necessary by face mask and self-inflating bag attached to oxygen or by tracheal intubation and self-inflating bag attached to oxygen.

Life-threatening injuries which impair ventilation are tension pneumothorax, open pneumothorax, massive haemothorax, flail chest with pulmonary contusion and cardiac tamponade.

The chest signs of a tension pneumothorax are deviation of the trachea away from the affected side, hyperresonant percussion note on the affected side and reduced breath sounds on the affected side. Decompress immediately by inserting a cannula through the second intercostal space in the mid-clavicular line on the affected side. This must be followed by placement of a chest drain.

Treat an open pneumothorax by placing a dressing over the injury and seal the dressing on three sides only to create a valve.

C   Circulation with aggressive volume replacement and haemorrhage control

Hypotension results in inadequate organ perfusion.

The commonest cause of hypotension in trauma is hypovolaemia due to haemorrhage. Successful outcome depends on early recognition of shock, restoration of volume and control of haemorrhage.

Signs of hypovolaemia are

- increase in heart rate
- cold, pale skin
- fall in urine output
- narrowed pulse pressure
- hypotension (late sign)

Have a low threshold of suspicion for bleeding and fluid replacement.

The pregnant patient will compensate for blood loss by reducing perfusion to the fetoplacental unit.

Pregnant women can lose up to 35% of their blood volume before signs of hypovolaemia develop. The fetus may be inadequately perfused although the mother's vital signs may be judged to be normal. The earliest sign of hypovolaemia may be fetal distress. If the mother is in shock there is an 80% risk of fetal mortality. 'Is the fetoplacental unit being perfused?'

Examples of blood loss
- fractured pelvis 3 l
- closed femoral fracture 1.5 l
- closed tibial fracture 500 ml

Place two large intravenous cannulae, take blood for FBC, U&Es, cross-match, coagulation screen, amylase and glucose.

If hypovolaemic replace fluid with warmed crystalloid, synthetic colloid or blood and blood products.

Continually assess response in heart rate, skin colour, urine output, level of consciousness and blood pressure to volume replacement. Beware of fluid overload if eclampsia or pre-eclampsia suspected.

Control haemorrhage by direct pressure or by operative intervention.

If failure to respond to volume replacement and haemorrhage control, consider massive blood loss, cardiogenic, anaphylactic, neurogenic or septic shock.

D   Disability – neurological assessment

Mini neurological assessment is by the AVPU method. Is the patient alert, responding to voice, pain or unresponsive?

Assess pupils and the presence of lateralizing signs.

Remember that fits may be due to eclampsia. Check blood pressure, reflexes, test for proteinuria and examine for oedema.

E   Exposure/environmental control

Completely undress patient to assess. Maintain body temperature by covering with warm blankets, maintaining warm room temperature and warming intravenous fluids.

Assess fetal well being and viability

Adequately resuscitate mother

Correct hypoxia and hypovolaemia.

Use ultrasound

The accuracy of ultrasound depends on the skill of the operator:

- to detect fetal heart and check rate
- to ascertain the number of babies and their positions
- to locate the position of the placenta and the amount of liquor
- to look for retroplacental bleeding or haematoma
- to detect an abnormal position of the fetus and free fluid in the abdominal cavity suggesting rupture of the uterus
- to detect damage to other structures, e.g. liver, spleen and kidneys
- to check for free fluid and blood

Trauma

Make decision whether to interrupt pregnancy either for fetal or maternal reasons

The fetus is most at risk during the four hours after trauma but there is a significant incidence of late abruption. Ascertain gestational age to assess fetal prognosis.

Indications for Caesarean section

- Fetal distress with a viable fetus.
- Placental abruption.
- Uterine rupture.
- An unstable pelvic or lumbosacral fracture with the patient in labour.
- Inadequate exposure during laparotomy for other abdominal trauma.
- Cardiac arrest.

Perimortem Caesarean section

Cardiopulmonary resuscitation (CPR) is ineffective unless left sided tilt is instituted and maintained. Even with tilt, aortocaval compression can compromise resuscitation. Emergency Caesarean section allows improvement in the venous return and should be performed after 5 min of unsuccessful, aggressive CPR in the correct position. It also reduces maternal oxygen consumption, makes ventilation easier and allows CPR to be carried out in the supine position.

Open cardiac massage should be considered early because of aortocaval compression.

A vertical midline incision and a midline incision into the uterus avoiding the bladder is used and the uterus is closed using a thick absorbable suture.

Maternal resuscitation should be continued throughout as there are recorded cases of late maternal survival.

Fetal prognosis after delivery at postmortem Caesarean section is very poor.

Assess and treat wounds to abdomen

Blunt trauma

The three commonest causes of blunt trauma in pregnancy are

- motor vehicle accident
- falls
- domestic violence

The pregnant uterus is a resilient organ and can tolerate severe pressure without rupturing. Rupture of the uterus may follow blunt trauma in association with seatbelts, although seatbelts reduce overall mortality in pregnant women.

The placenta and fetus are vulnerable despite the buffering effect of the amniotic fluid. The placenta because it is inelastic unlike the uterus and therefore is liable to shearing. There is a high chance of fetomaternal haemorrhage and a significant danger of abruption of the placenta. Fetal monitoring should be started early and the Kleihauer checked.

The incidence of domestic violence is increased in pregnancy, particularly direct blows to the abdomen.

Examination

The detection of intraperitoneal haemorrhage is even more difficult in the pregnant patient; 800 ml of blood needs to be present before reliable detection by ultrasound or X-rays.

The peritoneum in pregnancy has decreased sensitivity which may mask the signs of intraperitoneal injury.

The ultrasound focused abdominal sonography in trauma (FAST) test may be useful.

The indications for diagnostic peritoneal lavage are the same as for the non-pregnant patient.

Findings which increase the index of suspicion are:

- rib fractures, which suggest liver, spleen or kidney damage,
- pelvic fractures, which may be associated with massive retroperitoneal haemorrhage due to damage to dilated thin-walled pelvic veins, fracture of the fetal skull, damage to the bladder and rupture of the uterus.

Uterine rupture

This is uncommon and found in only 0.6% of pregnant trauma victims.

Maternal mortality is low – approximately 10% in severe injuries but fetal mortality approaches 100%.

Techniques to improve the chances of preserving the ruptured uterus and to control haemorrhage include:

(i) Medical

- Syntocinon.
- Ergometrine.
- Carboprost (Hemabate) 250 µg intramuscular or intramyometrial, maximum dose 2 mg.
- Vasopressin, subendometrial at bleeding site. Serial 1 ml injections. 5 IU (1 ml) vasopressin diluted in 19 ml of 0.9% sodium chloride. Injection should not be directly into a blood vessel.

(ii) Physical

- Direct pressure or bimanual compression.

(iii) Surgical

- Sound surgical technique, strong, thick sutures with generous bites of tissue.
- Ligation of the internal iliac artery in continuity – identify the bifurcation of the iliac artery and the ureter before tying the sutures.
- B-Lynch brace suture which compresses the uterus to achieve haemostasis.
- Hysterectomy – may be life-saving and needs to be performed without undue delay.

  Post-hysterectomy bleeding may be difficult to control and the use of a transvaginal pressure pack may be life-saving. A bag is placed in the pelvis and packed with gauze. The neck of the bag is brought through the vagina and the ends of the gauze packs are brought out through the vagina to facilitate later removal. A litre bag of fluid is attached to the neck of the bag to apply pressure.

Penetrating wounds

- Uncommon in Britain, much more common in the USA.
- Stab injury and gunshot wounds are most usual cause.
- Penetrating injuries above the uterine fundus tend to cause extensive gastro-intestinal and vascular damage.
- Penetrating injuries can cause uterine injury at any stage of pregnancy as the

uterine muscle and bony pelvis afford little protection against high velocity penetrating injuries.

- The uterus, fetus and liquor amnii reduce injury to the mother by absorbing energy and displacing bowel upwards and laterally.
- Gunshot wounds to the pregnant abdomen carry a high mortality for the fetus but a comparatively good prognosis for the mother.
- The incidence of visceral injuries in pregnant women with penetrating abdominal trauma is between 16 and 38% which compares with 80–90% in the general population with anterior abdominal gunshot wounds.
- Less than one in five women with a low velocity gunshot wound to the pregnant uterus will have extrauterine injury.
- The vast majority of gunshot wounds need to be explored.
- Meticulous examination of the abdominal contents is essential.

When to open the uterus

- If a bullet has entered the uterus and the fetus is alive and considered viable, Caesarean section is the safest course.
- If the fetus is dead and there is no obvious external bleeding from the uterine wall or intrauterine bleeding Caesarean section may occasionally be avoided: however in the vast majority of cases it will be safer to empty the uterus as delayed abruption after trauma is not uncommon.
- Caesarean hysterectomy may well need to be performed early in the presence of extensive uterine damage in association with other significant intra-abdominal injuries.
- Stab wounds generally cause injuries of lesser severity and fetal survival has followed repair of a uterine perforation.
- Fetal death is an indication for ending the pregnancy which will usually be by Caesarean section as trauma sufficient to kill the baby is likely to result in high chance of abruption, and the use of oxytocics on the recently traumatized uterus has a high risk of causing further uterine damage.

Assess fetomaternal haemorrhage

- In 30% of cases of severe trauma significant fetomaternal haemorrhage will occur.
- The Kleihauer test *must* be carried out in all cases of maternal trauma.
- All traumatized pregnant women should be given anti-D without waiting for the Kleihauer result.
- Further anti-D may need to be given in the light of the Kleihauer result.
- The Kleihauer test is sensitive, detecting a fetomaternal transfusion of less than 0.1 ml of fetal blood.
- A positive Kleihauer test is an indication for prolonged fetal monitoring.

Perform secondary survey and start definitive treatments

- Head to toe examination of the casualty including a log roll with the spine stabilized and a pelvic examination.
- Give particular attention to signs specific to the pregnant patient, e.g. vaginal bleeding, leakage of liquor and tenderness over the uterus.

When patient care optimized transfer if appropriate

Maternal or fetal conditions requiring treatment not available at the admitting centre necessitate transfer. The maternal condition should be optimized. If this requires transfer to another centre, and if this is best done without interruption of the pregnancy, the mother should be transferred before delivery. The centre of choice for further care is one which best meets maternal need but ideally one which meets the needs of both mother and fetus or newborn.

REFERENCE

Committee on Trauma (1997) *Advanced Trauma Life Support for Doctors.* American College of Surgeons.

ABNORMAL PATTERNS OF LABOUR

E. O'Donnell

Normal labour is characterized by regular uterine contractions, effacement and dilatation of the cervix, and descent of the presenting part.

Three abnormal patterns of labour can be identified when labour is plotted on a partogram. These are prolonged latent phase, primary dysfunctional labour, and secondary arrest.

The latent phase of labour begins with the onset of painful regular contractions and ends when the rate of cervical dilatation increases at the start of the accelerative phase of labour. The latent phase is defined as prolonged if it exceeds 6 h in a primipara or 4 h in a multipara. The incidence of this abnormal pattern of labour was found to be 3.5% in nulliparous women and was associated with a 10-fold increase in the frequency of Caesarean section.

Primary dysfunctional labour is defined as dilatation at a rate less than 1 cm/h in the active phase of labour. Incidence is 26% in nulliparous women.

Secondary arrest refers to a cessation in cervical dilatation after a period of normal active phase dilatation. Incidence is quoted as 6.3% in nulliparous women.

ACTION PLAN

1 **Ensure correct diagnosis of labour**

2 **Provide emotional and physical support according to the mother's individual needs**

3 **Assess progress of labour**

4 **Record all findings on the partogram**

5 **Assess the cause of slow progress by evaluation of the powers, passages and passenger**

6 **Correct slow progress with amniotomy and syntocinon**

7 **Use syntocinon with caution in the multiparous patient and with uterine scars**

8 **Beware of slow progress from 7–10 cm dilatation**

CONSULT OTHER TOPICS

Risk management (p. 185)

SUPPLEMENTARY INFORMATION

Ensure correct diagnosis of labour

The diagnosis of labour can of course only be made retrospectively. To diagnose labour there must be painful regular contractions, with associated dilatation and effacement.

Provide emotional and physical support according to the mother's individual needs

The active management policy proposed by O'Driscoll *et al.* (1984) and supported by recent trials has been shown to depend on a whole package of care which includes help and personal support in labour. Not all investigations have achieved a reduction in Caesarean section rate, however.

Robson *et al.* (1996) demonstrated a reduction in Caesarean section rate in primiparas at term from 7.5% to 2.4% using the following package of care.

- Careful attention to the accurate diagnosis of labour.
- Good personal support in labour.
- Artificial rupture of the membranes at 2 h if the rate of cervical dilatation was less than 1 cm/hour. (Recent studies have suggested that amniotomy alone is ineffective at correcting dystocia.)
- Oxytocin to augment labour after a further 2 hours if progress remained unsatisfactory.
- Two-hourly examinations if normal progress was occurring without syntocinon; 4-hourly vaginal examination after oxytocin was commenced unless indicated earlier.
- Pushing in the second stage only if the head was low and there was an urge to push.
- Oxytocin in the second stage after 1 hour if there was no descent of the head.
- Oxytocin for the second stage if there was no descent after 30 min of pushing.
- Women are encouraged to adopt whatever position they feel most comfortable, avoiding the supine position. Gravity and movement are considered to assist fetal descent and optimal fetal positioning.

Assess progress of labour

Assessment is by the strength and frequency of contractions, cervical effacement and dilatation, fetal position and station, and the presence of caput and moulding.

Record all findings on the partogram

The partogram is a structural representation of the progress of labour. This identifies that progress is maintained, ensures early recognition of problems and facilitates effective transfer of information to other care-givers.

Beware of slow progress from 7–10 cm dilatation

Slow progress during the 7–10 cm interval is associated with an increased incidence of instrumental deliveries and, as Davidson *et al.* (1976) highlighted, difficult instrumental delivery.

REFERENCES

Cardoza L, Gibb DMF, Studd JWW, Vasant RV and Cooper DJ (1982) Predictive value of cervimatric patterns in primigravidae. *Br. J. Obstet. Gynaecol.* **89**: 33–38.

Davidson AC, Weaver JB, Davies P and Pearson JF (1976) The relation between ease of forceps delivery and speed of cervical dilatation. *Br. J. Obstet. Gynaecol.* **83**: 279–283.

O'Driscoll K, Foley M and MacDonald D (1984) Active management of labour as an alternative to Cesarean section for dystocia. *Obstet. Gynecol.* **63**: 485–490.

Robson MS, Scudamore IW and Walsh SM (1996) Using the audit cycle to reduce Cesarean section rates. *Am. J. Obstet. Gynecol.* **174**: 199–205.

Abnormal Patterns of Labour

ABNORMAL PRESENTATIONS AND POSITIONS

BREECH

Richard Johanson and Charles Cox

DIAGNOSIS

The incidence is 3–4% at term, 16% at 32 weeks and 25% at 28 weeks. Breech may be diagnosed antenatally or not diagnosed until labour. If diagnosed, ultrasound should be used to assess whether the breech is extended (65%), flexed (25%) or footling (10%). Fetal abnormalities are increased in breech presentation and should be sought for antenatally.

ACTION PLAN

1 **For the breech diagnosed in pregnancy, consider method of delivery during the antenatal period**

2 **For the breech diagnosed in labour management will depend on the gestation, wishes of the mother and on clinical assessment of size and attitude of the fetus and maternal pelvis**

3 **Keep senior obstetrician informed**

4 **For elective Caesarean section**
- Ensure that the patient understands the concept of a trial of scar in a subsequent pregnancy (approximately 70% of women can be expected to achieve a vaginal delivery).
- Confirm that the baby is still a breech! Use ultrasound if there is any doubt.
- Deliver the baby as for an assisted breech/breech extraction. Forceps should be available to assist in delivering the fetal head.
- If the fetal head becomes trapped then the uterine incision may need to be extended either by extending into an inverted 'T' incision or better into a 'J' incision.

4 **For trial of vaginal breech**
- Confirm that the mother still wants a trial.
- Decide with the mother what analgesia she wishes to have, if any.
- An anaesthetist should be available immediately on site.
- Theatre facilities and paediatric cover should be immediately available.
- Fetal monitoring should be continuous.
- Amniotomy may be performed to accelerate labour. If the membranes rupture spontaneously then a vaginal examination should be carried out to exclude cord prolapse.

- Fetal blood sampling may be carried out from the buttock but if cardiotocographic evidence of fetal distress develops early in labour Caesarean section should be considered.
- Syntocinon is not contraindicated for delay but progress on the partogram should be at least as rapid as for a cephalic presentation.
- The management of the second stage should be supervised by an obstetrician experienced in breech delivery. If there is delay in the second stage there should be early recourse to Caesarean section.
- The basic principle is to avoid unnecessary interference. Hands off the breech!
- The breech should be allowed to descend to the pelvic floor without active pushing.
- The fetal anus should be seen over the fourchette before an episiotomy is performed.
- The breech will usually rotate to lie sacroanterior. If it tries to rotate posteriorly this should be prevented.
- Extended legs are delivered by flexion at the knee joint and extension at the hips.
- The body is supported and an attempt is made to bring down a loop of cord, rarely a short cord will prevent descent of the body.
- Further pushing brings the anterior shoulder scapular tip into view. A finger should now be run over the shoulder and down to the elbow to deliver the arm. The other shoulder will rotate anteriorly to allow a similar delivery of the other arm.
- The baby should be supported as the head engages. Delivery will often be accomplished by the Mauriceau–Smellie–Veit manouevre. Forceps should always be available. The guiding principle during delivery of the head is to control the delivery and avoid any sudden changes in intracranial pressure. The fetal head does not have time to adapt to the shape of the pelvis and forceps protect the head during delivery.
- If the head becomes extended, suprapubic pressure should guide the head into the pelvis.
- A weighted speculum placed in the vagina may aid delivery of the head, and this may also allow administration of oxygen to fetal nose and mouth.
- Symphisiotomy has been described but experience of this technique is likely to be limited. A urinary catheter is inserted and the urethra displaced laterally. The incision is made anteriorly and carried down to the ligament which is partially divided.

5   **Document procedure fully in notes with date, time, a signature and printed identification**

CONSULT OTHER TOPICS

Instrumental delivery – forceps (p. 75)
Instrumental delivery – ventouse (p. 78)
Neonatal resuscitation (p. 14)
Postpartum genital tract trauma (p. 104)

Abnormal Presentations and Positions

Premature labour (p. 110)
Risk management (p. 185)
Twins and multiple pregnancies (p. 122)

SUPPLEMENTARY INFORMATION

For the breech diagnosed in pregnancy, consider method of delivery during the antenatal period

- If associated complications, Caesarean section will usually be offered.
- The patient may be offered a choice of external cephalic version (ECV), elective Caesarean section or trial of vaginal delivery.
- External cephalic version should be carried out with the mother awake but starved and consented for Caesarean section, in the delivery suite with theatre facilities available. Cardiotocography should be performed before the procedure. The presentation of the fetus should be confirmed with ultrasound. Tocolysis (ritodrine) may be used as necessary. The breech and head are grasped and pressure exerted on the breech to push the baby around, head first.
- If the baby is thought to be large or the woman is of short stature, Caesarean section will be the safer option if ECV is declined. Consider use of maternal pelvimetry and ultrasound to estimate fetal weight.
- Many clinicians believe that the footling breech diagnosed antenatally should be delivered by Caesarean section.

For the breech diagnosed in labour management will depend on the gestation, wishes of the mother and on clinical assessment of size and attitude of the fetus and maternal pelvis

Many obstetricians feel that if there has not been opportunity for comprehensive antenatal assessment and discussion, Caesarean section is the preferred option from the risk management point of view. However there is no evidence to suggest that Caesarean section is preferable to vaginal delivery for the premature breech.

For trial of vaginal breech

- Decide with the mother what analgesia she wishes to have if any.

  An epidural anaesthetic is particularly recommended for multiparous women to prevent them pushing too soon and causing entrapment of the head by the undilated cervix (this is especially so if the breech is premature and the mother is permitted to labour).
- The body is supported and an attempt is made to bring down a loop of cord; rarely a short cord will prevent descent of the body.

  In any manoeuvre, the body is controlled by the pelvifemoral grip, taking care to avoid pressure on the abdomen which may lead to liver damage.

SYSTEMATIC REVIEWS

Hofmeyr GJ (1999) External cephalic version for breech presentation before term (Cochrane Review). *The Cochrane Library*, Issue 2. Update Software, Oxford.

Reviewers' conclusions: *External cephalic version before term does not appear to improve pregnancy outcomes.*

Hofmeyr GJ and Kulier R (1999) External cephalic version for breech presentation at term (Cochrane Review). *The Cochrane Library*, Issue 2, 1999. Update Software, Oxford.

Reviewers' conclusions: *Attempting cephalic version at term appears to reduce the chance of non-cephalic births and Caesarean section. There is not enough evidence to assess any risks of external cephalic version at term.*

Hofmeyr GJ (1999) External cephalic version facilitation for breech presentation at term (Cochrane Review). *The Cochrane Library*, Issue 2. Update Software, Oxford.

Reviewers' conclusions: *Routine tocolysis appeares to reduce the failure rate of external cephalic version at term. Although promising, there is not enough evidence to evaluate the use of fetal acoustic stimulation in midline fetal spine positions. There is not enough evidence to evaluate the use of epidural analgesia or transabdominal amnioinfusion for external cephalic version at term.*

Hofmeyr GJ and Hannah ME (1999) Planned Caesarean section for term breech delivery (Cochrane Review). *The Cochrane Library*, Issue 2. Update Software, Oxford.

Reviewers' conclusions: *There is not enough evidence to evaluate the use of a policy of planned Caesarean section for breech presentation. A large Canadian trial addressing this question is currently underway.*

Hofmeyr GJ and Kulier R (1999) Expedited versus conservative approaches for vaginal delivery in breech presentation (Cochrane Review). *The Cochrane Library*, Issue 2. Update Software, Oxford.

Reviewers' conclusions: *There is not enough evidence to evaluate the effects of expedited vaginal breech delivery.*

Hofmeyr GJ and Kulier R (1999)Cephalic version by postural management for breech presentation (Cochrane Review). *The Cochrane Library*, Issue 2. Update Software, Oxford.

Reviewers' conclusions: *There is not enough evidence to evaluate the use of postural management for breech presentation.*

Renfrew MJ and Neilson JP (1994) Cochrane Database of Systematic Reviews 03087 4 Oct 1993, published through *Cochrane update on disk*, Disk issue 1. Update Software, Oxford.

BROW

DIAGNOSIS

- Usually made in labour but may be made antenatally by ultrasound.
- Abdominal palpation may give a clue because on palpation of the head the occiput will be felt higher than the synciput on the same side as the back.
- On vaginal examination a hard, high, rounded part presents, the bregma occupying the centre of the dilating cervix. The frontal suture, the anterior fontanelle and the orbital region may be found. The nose mouth and chin will not be felt.

ACTION PLAN

1 **Normal delivery is not possible for a normal size baby and a Caesarean section should be carried out**

2 **Premature babies may deliver as a brow**

3 **In patients who refuse Caesarean section, use the technique of disempacting the head in labour under ritodrine relaxation and bimanually flexing the head with one hand in the vagina and the other on the abdomen. This is done under ultrasound control.** Flexion of the head may be encouraged by the use of the Ventouse

COMPOUND

Compound presentation includes cases of cephalic presentation where one or more limbs present with the head and also breech presentation when one or more arms present with the breech. Commonly occurs in prematurity.

DIAGNOSIS

- By feeling a foot or hand alongside or in front of the presenting part.
- A hand can be differentiated from a foot by feeling for the thumb or feeling a heel of the foot.

ACTION PLAN

1 **Expectant management unless there is an associated cord prolapse**

2 **Active treatment only required if cord prolapse or delay in the first or second stages**

FACE

DIAGNOSIS

- Usually made in labour, often late in labour.
- Often confused with a breech presentation because of the soft tissues.
- Findings include palpable jaws, nose, cheek bones and orbital ridges.

ACTION PLAN

1 **If the chin is towards the pubis (mentoanterior) then the baby can often deliver normally.** However an episiotomy is necessary

2 **The progress of labour should be monitored carefully. Slow progress should lead to Caesarean section**

3 **If forceps delivery is considered then the head must be confirmed to be fully engaged**

4 **If the chin is towards the sacrum (mentoposterior) then Caesarean section should be performed**

5 **In patients who refuse Caesarean section, use the technique of disempacting the head in labour under ritodrine relaxation and bimanually flexing the head with one hand in the vagina and the other on the abdomen. This is done under ultrasound control**

OCCIPITOPOSTERIOR POSITION

This is very common, occurring in 20% of labouring women.

DIAGNOSIS

- Flattening of the abdomen (scaphoid or boat-shaped abdomen).
- The fetal back is difficult to define and limbs may be felt anteriorly.
- The head may be difficult to feel abdominally.
- The fetal heart is usually heard better towards the flanks.
- Vaginal examination reveals a high deflexed head.

ACTION PLAN

1   **Ensure adequate uterine activity if a primiparous woman, by the judicious use of syntocinon**

2   **Ensure adequate analgesia**
- An epidural is helpful to reduce pushing before full dilatation.

3   **Syntocinon may need to be started in the second stage of labour to encourage rotation of the head in the primiparous woman**

4   **The partogram may give the diagnosis in the primiparous woman by demonstrating secondary arrest of labour.** This is usually before full dilatation. Multiparous women usually reach full dilatation and are at risk of uterine rupture from unrecognized cephalopelvic disproportion

5   **Assisted delivery is frequently required for persistent occipitoposterior positions**

6   **Ventouse is the preferred method of delivery and the OP cup should be used**
- Alternatives are to deliver the baby's head face to pubes if the head is well down, to do a manual rotation of the head then complete the delivery by forceps (this procedure requires adequate analgesia and disempaction of the head before rotation can be carried out) or rotational forceps delivery with the Kiellands forceps (this procedure should only be carried out by someone with extensive experience of the procedure).

7   **Caesarean section is often indicated as there is relative cephalopelvic disproportion**
- This procedure may be difficult as the head may well be deeply engaged and tears may occur in the lower segment. It is helpful

for the operator or the assistant to disempact the head from below before the abdomen is opened. Pushing posteriorly in the vagina will only cause further deflexion – push at 12 o'clock to encourage flexion.

TRANSVERSE/OBLIQUE LIE

Instead of the baby lying longitudinally, the baby lies transversley or obliquely.

DIAGNOSIS

- Abnormal shape of the uterus with the fundus broader and lower than would be expected from the gestation.
- No fetal pole in the pelvis.

1 **Antenatally**
- Exclude placenta praevia or any other structural problem which would preclude engagement of the fetal head, such as a pelvic tumour. This can be reliably detected by ultrasound, especially transvaginal.
- Recurrent unstable lies should be admitted at 37 weeks' gestation.
- An attempt at external cephalic version (ECV) can be made and if the lie remains cephalic induction of labour should be considered (stabilizing induction).

2 **At delivery**
- Caesarean section should be carried out if the lie remains transverse despite attempted ECV.
- A traditional transverse lower segment incision is usually employed but if the fetal back is inferior and access to the fetal head and limbs compromised then an upper segment vertical incision can be used.
- If difficulty is encountered during the delivery then the uterine incision can be extended using the 'J' incision or the inverted 'T'.

ACUTE ABDOMINAL PAIN

It is important to make an early diagnosis so that life-threatening causes may be quickly treated. Acute abdominal pain in pregnancy, especially if associated with uterine tenderness and/or signs of shock or hypovolaemia must be assumed to be due to placental abruption until proved otherwise. Pain may be pregnancy related, exacerbated by pregnancy or unrelated to pregnancy. Surgical procedures are well tolerated in pregnancy and where indicated surgery should be performed early.

ACTION PLAN

1 **Airway**
   - Assess.
   - Maintain patency.
   - Apply oxygen 15 l/min via tight fitting face mask with reservoir bag.
   - Attach pulse oximeter to patient.
   - Call anaesthetist.

   Breathing
   - Assess.
   - Assist.
   - Protect airway.

   Circulation
   - Assess.
   - CPR.
   - Tilt to left.
   - Put on ECG and BP monitor.
   - Treat peri-arrest arrhythmias.
   - I.v. access, send bloods for FBC, U&Es, LFTs, glucose, amylase and G&S or cross-match, start i.v.i.
   - Treat hypotension.

2 **Check fetal heart and if delivery needed consider timing and method**

3 **Assess cause of pain and treat specifically – consider turning off epidural infusion. Remember placental abruption!**

4 **If placental abruption, pre-eclampsia or ruptured uterus suspected call senior obstetric help**

5 **Call for help from other specialties (general surgeons or anaesthetists) in the assessment and treatment of non-pregnancy causes**

6 **Keep record chart to include pulse, BP, RR, SaO$_2$, temperature, FH and treatments given**

7 **Document examination, investigation and diagnosis clearly in notes, with time, date, a signature and printed identification and inform consultant obstetrician if appropriate**

CONSULT OTHER TOPICS

Airway obstruction (p. 1)
Cardiopulmonary resuscitation (p. 8)
Eclampsia, pre-eclampsia, HELLP, fatty liver and hepatic rupture (p.66)
Hypotension (p. 150)
Massive obstetric haemorrhage – antepartum (p. 88)
Peri-arrest arrhythmias (p. 16)
Respiratory emergencies (p. 20)
Risk management (p. 185)
Sickle cell crisis (p. 165)
Uterine rupture (p. 125)

SUPPLEMENTARY INFORMATION

Assess cause of pain and treat specifically

Causes related to pregnancy

- Abruptio placentae either revealed or concealed. Remember trauma – a comparatively trivial injury may result in abruption of the placenta which may be delayed for some time after the injury.
- Pre-eclampsia (PET) and HELLP leading to pain in the right upper quadrant due to stretching of the capsule of the liver.
- Spontaneous rupture of the uterus usually following classical Caesarean section or uterine surgery. Pain of uterine rupture will break through epidural analgesia. Spontaneous uterine rupture is unlikely unless in labour.
- Braxton-Hicks contractions and fetal movements.
- Pressure from the enlarging uterus.
- Pubic diastasis causing lower abdominal pain and tenderness.

Causes exacerbated by pregnancy

- Heartburn from gastrointestinal reflux.
- Gall bladder disease is increased in pregnancy.
- Urinary tract infections, bacteruria, pyelonephritis, acute cystitis.
- Musculoskeletal pain.

Non-pregnancy causes of pain

- Appendicitis is more difficult to diagnose because of the frequency of abdominal pain in pregnancy. The site of pain tends to be higher and more lateral, because the appendix is displaced by the gravid uterus.
- Acute cholecystitis.
- Acute pancreatitis is rare but has a mortality of greater than 10%.
- Peptic ulcer is uncommon.
- Inflammatory bowel disease may improve with pregnancy.
- Renal stones are uncommon in pregnancy because of dilatation of the renal tract.
- Malignant pain.
- Porphyria is uncommon.
- Rupture of the inferior epigastric artery, usually due to coughing.
- Sickle cell crisis.
- Splenic or renal artery rupture is rare.

Pregnancy related causes of abdominal pain in early pregnancy

- Abortion.
- Molar pregnancy.
- Ectopic pregnancy.
- Accidents to ovarian cysts.
- Acute retention of urine due to retroversion of the uterus, incarcerated fibroids or ovarian cysts.
- Stretching of the round ligaments.
- Degeneration of a fibroid.
- Complications of amniocentesis.

Call for help from other specialties (general surgeons or anaesthetists) in the assessment and treatment of non-pregnancy causes

It is inappropriate for an obstetrician in training to seek the opinion of a general surgeon. Discussion should be at consultant level.

AMNIOTIC FLUID EMBOLISM

The Report on Confidential Enquiries into maternal deaths in the UK 1994–1996 reports amniotic fluid embolism as the third leading cause of direct deaths. The condition occurs when a bolus of amniotic fluid is released during contractions into the maternal circulation. It has cardiorespiratory effects as it becomes trapped in the maternal pulmonary circulation and it causes disseminated intra-vascular coagulation (DIC).

ACTION PLAN

1 **Suspect**

2 **Call for help including senior obstetrician and anaesthetist**

3 **Airway**
- Assess.
- Maintain patency.
- Apply oxygen 15 l/min via tight fitting face mask with reservoir bag.
- Attach pulse oximeter to patient.
- Consider early tracheal intubation if cardiovascular collapse or respiratory distress.

Breathing
- Assess.
- Ventilate with 100% oxygen if respiratory distress.
- May need positive end expiratory pressure to ventilate adequately.

Circulation
- Assess for signs of circulation and BP.
- CPR.
- Tilt to left.
- Put on ECG and BP monitor.
- Treat peri-arrest arrhythmias.
- Secure two large bore i.v. cannulae, send FBC, clotting studies and cross-match 6 units, run i.v.i.

4 **Treat hypotension by replacement of intravascular volume with synthetic colloid and blood and increments of ephedrine 3 mg i.v. titrated against BP**

5 **Assess central venous pressure which reveals an initial rise due to acute pulmonary hypertension and eventually a decrease due to haemorrhage**

6 **Request CXR and V/Q scan**

7 **Consult haematologist and with advice treat DIC with whole blood if available, fresh frozen plasma, platelets and cryoprecipitate**

8 **Discuss heparin therapy with haematologist**

9 **If undelivered, deliver immediately – surgical if necessary**

10 **Control uterine haemorrhage if delivered with uterine massage and i.v. oxytocics, ergometrine, haemabate and aprotinin**

11 **If unresponsive consider exploration for retained placenta or genital tract trauma**

12 **Consider differential diagnosis**

13 **Transfer to ICU for continued supportive therapy**

14 **Consider the use of salbutamol, aminophylline, dopamine, hydrocortisone and diuretics in joint management with intensivists**

15 **Keep a record to include pulse, BP, CVP, RR, SaO$_2$, FH and treatments given**

16 **Document in notes concisely and chronologically, with time, date, a signature and printed identification**

CONSULT OTHER TOPICS

SUPPLEMENTARY INFORMATION

Suspect

- Amniotic fluid embolism usually presents during the latter part of the first stage of labour.
- Symptoms include chills, shivering, sweating, anxiety, coughing.
- Signs are respiratory distress manifest as cyanosis, tachypnoea, bronchospasm or even frank pulmonary oedema, cardiovascular collapse manifest as hypotension, tachycardia, arrhythmias and cardiac arrest.
- Convulsions may occur secondary to cerebral ischaemia.
- DIC may quickly develop.

Request CXR and V/Q scan

CXR may show enlargement of the right atrium and ventricle, a prominent proximal artery and pulmonary oedema.

Consider differential diagnosis

- Pulmonary thromboembolism.
- Air embolism.
- Aspiration pneumonitis.
- Eclamptic convulsions.
- Local anaesthetic toxicity.
- Haemorrhagic shock.
- Left heart failure.

BORN BEFORE ARRIVAL

Born before arrival refers to an intended delivery outside the hospital. The following care is administered before arrival at the hospital. Transfer of mother and baby to hospital is usual. If both are well, however, they may remain at home.

ACTION PLAN

1 **Check condition of mother**
   - Airway.
   - Breathing.
   - Circulation.

2 **Check condition of the baby – if necessary resuscitate**

3 **Check to see if the placenta has been delivered and the uterus is well contracted**

4 **If continued bleeding rub up a contraction and check the genital tract for lacerations**
   - Administer an oxytocic if available.

5 **If the placenta is obviously incomplete and heavy bleeding continues, do a vaginal examination to check whether there is a piece of placenta sitting in the cervix. If there is, remove it**

6 **There is no hurry to ligate and cut the cord. This can safely be delayed until appropriate equipment is at hand**

7 **If the cord has snapped, ligate it at least 5 cm from the baby**

8 **If the placenta is undelivered, rub up a contraction and administer an oxytocic if available**

9 **Deliver the placenta as normal by controlled cord traction**

10 **If the uterus is inverted, attempt immediate manual replacement**

11 **Dry baby and wrap up warmly**

12 **Document in notes with times, date, a signature and printed identification condition of mother and baby and management**

CONSULT OTHER TOPICS

Hypotension (p. 150)
Inverted uterus (p. 85)
Massive obstetric haemorrhage – postpartum (p. 95)
Neonatal resuscitation (p. 14)
Peri-arrest arrhythmias (p. 16)
Respiratory emergencies (p. 20)
Retained placenta (p. 116)

SUPPLEMENTARY INFORMATION

Check condition of mother

- Unplanned births at home are more likely to be complicated by precipitate labour, breech presentation and postpartum haemorrhage.
- Blood loss should be estimated and the haemoglobin checked if the patient is unbooked or has not had a recent one carried out.
- The blood group must be ascertained as anti-D may be required.
- If the patient is unbooked all the routine screening tests should be carried out and the patient considered to be at higher risk of blood-borne infections.

Born Before Arrival

CAESAREAN HYSTERECTOMY

Richard Johanson and Charles Cox

Caesarean hysterectomy is defined as the removal of the pregnant or recently pregnant uterus due to complications of delivery. 'Peripartum hysterectomy' includes Caesarean and postpartum hysterectomy. Caesarean hysterectomy can be an emergency or planned procedure.

1 **The indications for an emergency Caesarean hysterectomy are the following life-threatening conditions**
   - Haemorrhage, often atonic.
   - Ruptured uterus after previous Caesarean section or neglected or mismanaged labour.
   - Placental problems, particularly placenta accreta.
   - Sepsis due to prolonged rupture of the membranes.
   - Ectopic pregnancy occurring in the cornua of the uterus or in the cervix.
   - Expanding pelvic haematomas following termination of pregnancy.

2 **Airway**
   - Assess.
   - Maintain patency.
   - Apply oxygen 15 l/min via tight fitting face mask with reservoir bag.
   - Attach pulse oximeter to patient.
   - Call anaesthetist.

   Breathing
   - Assess.
   - Ventilate.
   - Protect airway.

   Circulation
   - Assess pulse and BP.
   - CPR.
   - Put on ECG and automatic BP monitor.
   - Treat peri-arrest arrhythmias.
   - I.v. access (two large bore cannulae), send bloods for FBC and cross-match; consider clotting studies if massive haemorrhage, start i.v.i.
   - Treat hypotension.

3 **Call senior obstetrician, resident anaesthetist and paediatrician**

4 **Take informed consent for Caesarean hysterectomy in all cases of massive postpartum haemorrhage, cases of suspected ruptured uterus and consider in cases of placenta praevia. Inform the patient's partner**

5 **Adequate amounts of blood should be immediately available – hasten cross-match and collection of cross-matched**

blood. **Have supplies of Group 0 negative blood readily available**

6 **Insert urinary catheter**

7 **Operative technique**
- A midline incision may be preferable to facilitate access to the rest of the abdomen and to carry out a classical Caesarean section in cases of planned Caesarean hysterectomy.
- Subtotal hysterectomy reduces haemorrhage and the risk of damage to the bladder and ureter.
- Take rapid control of major blood vessels.
- Control retrograde bleeding from severed vessels.
- Transfix all pedicles as loosening of the sutures may occur after bleeding settles.
- Carefully control collateral blood vessels by ligation.
- Use of local tourniquet, e.g. rubber catheters or intravenous tubing around the uterus if bleeding heavy.
- Manual compression of the aorta may be used to reduce bleeding while haemostasis is achieved.
- Ligation of internal iliac vessels may be necessary.
- Use pressure packs to control venous haemorrhage that occurs posthysterectomy.
- Salpingo-oophorectomy may be necessary in cases of broad ligament haematoma or bleeding from the ovarian vessels in approximately 15–20% of cases.

8 **Be aware of postoperative complications**

9 **Keep record chart to include pulse, BP, RR, SaO$_2$, treatments given and methods used**

10 **Record clearly in notes with times, date, a signature and printed identification and inform consultant obstetrician if not already present**

CONSULT OTHER CHAPTERS

SUPPLEMENTARY INFORMATION

The indications for an emergency Caesarean hysterectomy are the following life-threatening conditions

Indications for non-emergency Caesarean hysterectomy are:

- haemorrhage, often atonic
- ruptured uterus after previous Caesarean section or neglected or mismanaged labour
- placental problems, particularly placenta accreta
- sepsis due to prolonged rupture of the membranes
- ectopic pregnancy occurring in the cornua of the uterus or in the cervix
- expanding pelvic haematomas following termination of pregnancy
- multiple previous Caesarean sections
- uterine leiomyomas
- cervical neoplasia
- certain benign gynaecological conditions

Call senior obstetrician, resident anaesthetist and paediatrician

Caesarean hysterectomy is a procedure which should be performed by a senior obstetrician.

Operative technique

Take rapid control of major blood vessels by manual compression of the uterine vessels or the use of myomectomy clamps. Myomectomy clamps may not be part of the hysterectomy set and a specific request may have to be made to theatre.

Be aware of postoperative complications

Postoperative complications include:

- continued bleeding requiring re-laparotomy
- damage to the bladder and ureter
- infection
- ileus
- thromboembolic phenomena

CAESAREAN SECTION – COMPLICATIONS

Richard Johanson and Charles Cox

ACTION PLAN

1 Consider general anaesthetic and spinal/epidural block complications

2 Anticipate problems of access

3 Anticipate difficulty in delivering the baby

4 Control haemorrhage

5 Be aware of damage to other structures

6 Manage unexpected findings

7 Prevent infection

CONSULT OTHER TOPICS

Caesarean hysterectomy (p. 52)
Massive obstetric haemorrhage – DIC (p. 92)
Massive obstetric haemorrhage – postpartum (p. 95)
Puerperal sepsis, septicaemia and septic shock (p. 113)
Spinals and epidurals – high spinal anaesthesia (p. 169)
Spinals and epidurals – local anaesthetic toxicity (p. 171)

SUPPLEMENTARY INFORMATION

Anticipate problems of access

If previous surgery or scarring

- Ensure appropriate adequate incision.
- Excise a previous scar and ensure access by adequate dissection of the sheath off the underlying muscle. This may be time-consuming!
- The bladder may well be hitched up, especially after a previous Caesarean section. If the bladder is opened it is only a problem if it goes unrecognized and is left unrepaired.
- Ensure the incision is large enough to insert your hand and deliver the baby's head.

If anterior placenta praevia

This may be best managed by a vertical incision in the uterus to avoid very large vessels, but if the blood vessels are not particularly big a routine lower segment Caesarean section can be performed, a hand swept around the placenta to separate it from the uterine wall and the presenting part grasped and delivered. Part of the placenta may need to be delivered before the fetus.

If fibroids

May be present in the lower segment and may impede engagement of the head or cause a malposition. It is unwise to attempt a myomectomy at the time of Caesarean section and a higher vertical incision to avoid the fibroid is likely to be safer.

If previous major bowel or bladder surgery

Caesarean section may be made more difficult due to adhesions but even after procedures such as augmentation cystoplasty, delivery is often surprisingly straightforward. If the bladder is adherent and cannot be separated a midline incision to avoid damage to the ureters can be made in the bladder. A senior obstetrician should be consulted and urological assistance requested as indicated. The ureters should be identified and if necessary, catheterized.

Anticipate difficulty in delivering the baby

If the head is deeply engaged

The head should be disempacted before the Caesarean section is started. It is much easier to do it then than during the procedure.

If there is prematurity or placenta praevia

Minimize the risk by making sure there is adequate access through the abdominal incision and that the correct uterine incision is selected, e.g if there is a major degree of placenta praevia and the fetus is a premature breech then a classical Caesarean section is to be preferred. If fully dilated, cut high to avoid bladder.

If the fetus is transverse

The position of the head should be determined so that the feet may be grasped when the uterus is opened. The lie of the fetus should have been determined by ultrasound if there was any doubt.

If the incision is inadequate and it is not possible to deliver the baby without the use of undue force the incision should be extended. This is best done by extending the incision upwards from the lateral end of the uterine incision to produce a 'J' shaped incision. An alternative is to carry out an inverted 'T' incision. The theoretical disadvantage to this incision is that it may be more likely to rupture in a subsequent pregnancy.

Control haemorrhage

Consider exteriorizing uterus from the abdominal cavity. Ask the anaesthetist first and tell the patient if she is awake! Risk of air embolism may be increased.

Temporary control of haemorrhage can be obtained by myomectomy clamps being placed over the uterine arteries or by direct digital pressure over the arteries.

If the bleeding is uncontrollable then direct pressure can be applied to the aorta. Summon a senior obstetrician.

If atonic uterine muscle, compress uterus and administer a further dose of an oxytocic and continue with a syntocinon drip. Carboprost may be injected directly into the uterine muscle.

If the placenta is adherent and there is no significant bleeding the placenta can be left to absorb. Attempts to remove a morbidly adherent placenta may damage the uterine wall and cause severe haemorrhage and are associated with an increased risk of infection.

Bleeding commonly occurs from extension of the uterine incision at the angles causing damage to the uterine vessels. If the uterine artery is identified it can be ligated in continuity, otherwise deep sutures should be placed just lateral to the edge of the incision.

Early consideration should be given to hysterectomy in cases of severe haemorrhage after Caesarean section as delay leads to a significantly increased mortality.

Secondary postpartum haemorrhage can occasionally be severe and presumably arises from erosion into a blood vessel, possibly due to local infection. Laparotomy may be required and the patient should be consented for hysterectomy.

Be aware of damage to other structures

Bladder

As long as the damage is identified and repaired, long-term problems are very uncommon. The damage can be repaired with catgut or a synthetic absorbable material. The sutures and technique employed however should be those with which the operator is comfortable. The bladder should be on catheter drainage for 5 days at least, and antibiotics continued. A senior obstetrician should be consulted at the time of the damage.

Bowel

It is easy to incise into small bowel during entry into the peritoneum and bowel adjacent to the incision should be inspected. The defect can usually be simply closed with one layer of absorbable *or* non-absorbable suture. The consultant obstetrician should be consulted and if necessary a general surgeon. The patient should be kept on a 'soft' diet for a few days.

Ureter

The ureter is at risk when there is troublesome haemorrhage from the angles of the incision and wide deep haemostatic sutures are employed. Patients do not immediately die of ureteric injury but may die from haemorrhage. Haemorrhage control therefore takes priority! Call a senior member of the obstetric staff who will usually consult a urologist if ureteric damage is confirmed.

Broad ligament haematomas may be controlled by direct compression or it may be necessary to open up the leaves of the ligament to identify bleeding points and identify the ureters before the insertion of sutures.

Tearing of the rectus muscles may cause troublesome haemorrhage and on occasion it may be necessary to divide the recti transversely to improve access. Cutting diathermy may be useful when dividing the recti, but bleeding from tears is likely to be better dealt with by suturing the bleeding points. The muscle layer beneath the sheath should be drained and the sheath closed with a strong long-lasting suture.

Manage unexpected findings

Ovarian masses

If suspicious of malignancy call senior clinician for advice and take a biopsy. Dermoid cysts can be enucleated in the normal way. Simple looking cysts may be excised but the rule is to be as conservative as possible and for definitive surgery to be carried out as an elective procedure.

Fibroids

Comparatively common and usually an incidental finding. They should not be removed unless causing distortion of the uterine cavity leading to difficulty with haemorrhage control.

Dehiscence of a previous lower segment Caesarean section scar

This should be noted and repaired.

Torsion of the uterus

Identify the bladder and gently rotate the uterus back to the neutral position.

Prevent infection

Systematic reviews show that antibiotic prophylaxis reduces infection after Caesarean section by two thirds to three quarters. Both ampicillin and first generation cephalosporins have similar efficacy. Infection can occur after failure to adequately drain the uterus after Caesarean section when cervical stenosis is present. At every Caesarean section a finger should be passed through the cervix to allow free passage of lochia.

SYSTEMATIC REVIEWS

Enkin MW and Wilkinson C (1999) Uterine exteriorization versus intraperitoneal repair at Caesarean section (Cochrane Review). *The Cochrane Library*, Issue 2. Update Software, Oxford.

Reviewers' conclusions: *There is not enough evidence to evaluate the routine use of exteriorization of the uterus for repair of the uterine incision.*

Enkin MW and Wilkinson C (1999) Manual removal of placenta at Caesarean section (Cochrane Review). *The Cochrane Library*, Issue 2. Update Software, Oxford.

Reviewers' conclusions: *The evidence suggests that manual removal of placenta at Caesarean section may do more harm than good, by increasing maternal blood loss and increasing the risk of infection.*

Hopkins L and Smaill F (1999) Antibiotic prophylaxis regimens and drugs for Caesarean section (Cochrane Review). *The Cochrane Library*, Issue 2. Update Software, Oxford.

Reviewers' conclusions: *Both ampicillin and first generation cephalosporins have similar efficacy in reducing postoperative endometritis. There does not appear to be added benefit in utilizing a more broad spectrum agent or a multiple dose regimen. There is a need for an appropriately designed randomized trial to test the optimal timing of administration (immediately after the cord is clamped versus preoperative).*

Smaill F and Hofmeyr GJ (1999) Antibiotic prophylaxis for ceasarean section (Cochrane Review). *The Cochrane Library*, Issue 2. Update Software, Oxford.

Reviewers' conclusions: *The reduction of endometritis by two thirds to three quarters justifies a policy of administering prophylactic antibiotics to women undergoing elective or non-elective Caesarean section.*

CERVICAL STENOSIS IN LABOUR

Scarring to the cervix may follow operations to the cervix such as large loop excision of the transformation zone and cold knife conization. The cervix fails to dilate despite good uterine acitivity. The incidence of this complication is low but if unrecognised can lead to fetal distress and, in the multiparous patient especially, to rupture of the uterus.

ACTION PLAN

1 **Suspect**

2 **Diagnose – palpate cervix and identify cervical os**

3 **Consult an experienced obstetrician**

4 **Break through the area of scarring with a finger, forceps or a knife** – the cervix should then dilate rapidly

CONSULT OTHER TOPICS

Massive obstetric haemorrhage – antepartum (p. 88)
Massive obstetric haemorrhage – postpartum (p. 95)
Uterine rupture (p. 125)

SUPPLEMENTARY INFORMATION

Suspect

Risk factors are previous surgery or treatments to the cervix. The history may have to be by direct enquiry as patients often forget procedures such as a large loop excision of the transformation zone.

Suspect if the cervical os fails to dilate despite good contractions, especially in a multiparous patient.

Suspect if unable to identify the cervical os or to insert a finger through it.

Diagnose – palpate cervix and identify cervical os

Attempt to identify the os. There may be nothing obvious to palpate or, more commonly, a dimple will be felt. It may not be possible to pass the tip of a finger or a forcep through this dimple easily. A thinned cervix tightly applied to the fetal head may be mistaken for the fetal membranes with resulting increased risk of uterine damage either from rupture or trauma to the cervix from attempts to rupture the membranes.

Caution: Occasionally, the diagnosis may not be made, for example in the case of an elective Caesarean section, and difficulty is experienced in identifying the cervical canal from above. It is essential that there is a conduit for lochia to drain as haeatometra is certain to occur. The abdomen should not be closed until this has been achieved. This may require a simultaneous approach from above and below.

Break through the area of scarring with a finger, forceps or a knife

Once the dimple of the os has been identified, try to push a finger through the dimple. If unsuccessful, use the digitally guided tips of a pair of forceps such as Kocher's forceps to press firmly against the dimple and open the tips.

Occasionally, it may be necessary to directly incise over the mid portion of the cervix if no dimple is palpable. Once a superficial incision has been made in a cruciate manner over the presumed site of the os a finger should be used to break through the scar tissue. The patient should be in full lithotomy position and be provided with adequate analgesia. Once the scar tissue has been broken down or divided, the cervix can be expected to dilate rapidly and delivery to proceed apace.

Bleeding from the cervix is rarely a problem, but if it occurs it can be simply controlled with sutures.

CORD PROLAPSE

Richard Johanson and Charles Cox

Cord prolapse is defined as prolapse of the umbilical cord past the presenting part in the presence of ruptured membranes or active labour.

ACTION PLAN

1 **Suspect**

2 **Diagnose by palpating cord – consider occult prolapse**

3 **Do not panic – rushing makes other accidents more likely**

4 **Summon senior obstetrician, resident anaesthetist and paediatrician**

5 **Replace the cord above the presenting part if the patient is remote from the place of delivery**

6 **Elevate the presenting part to reduce pressure on cord**
- Fill the bladder via a Foley catheter to a volume of 400–750 ml. The presenting part is lifted out of the pelvis by the bladder.

7 **Monitor fetal heart rate by cardiotocograph**

8 **Deliver the baby if alive**
- Ventouse or forceps if cervix fully dilated.
- Caesarean section.

9 **If not alive await normal vaginal delivery**

10 **Keep record chart to include FH, treatments given and methods**

11 **Document clearly in notes, with date, time, a signature and printed identification and inform consultant obstetrician**

CONSULT OTHER TOPICS

Abnormal presentations and positions – breech (p. 34)
Instrumental delivery – forceps (p. 75)
Instrumental delivery – ventouse (p. 78)
Neonatal resuscitation (p. 14)
Premature labour (p. 110)
Risk management (p. 185)
Twins and multiple pregnancies (p. 122)

SUPPLEMENTARY INFORMATION

Suspect

Risk factors are low birth weight, premature labour, breech presentation, multiparity and being a second born twin.

Diagnose by palpating cord

An occult prolapse of the cord may manifest itself by fetal distress. Assess whether the cord is pulsating. If not use ultrasound to visualize the fetal heart to ascertain fetal viability.

Do not panic

There is no panic if the presenting part is elevated and there is no fetal distress.

Elevate the presenting part to reduce pressure on cord

- By filling the bladder via a Foley catheter. The quantity of saline needed is determined by the appearance of the distended bladder above the pubis. The balloon is then inflated, the catheter clamped and the drainage tubing and urine bag are attached and secured. A full bladder also seems to inhibit uterine contractions and pressure is taken off the cord.

Alternatives are:

- manual elevation of the presenting part above the pelvic inlet to relieve cord compression,
- knee–chest position or Trendelenburg (head down) position with manual elevation of the presenting part above the pelvic brim to relieve compression on the cord.

Deliver the baby

If the cervix is fully dilated and the head is engaged consider delivery by forceps or Ventouse.

If vaginal delivery is not possible proceed to emergency Caesarean section with normal, safe anaesthetic and surgical practice. If the bladder has been distended it should be deflated before entering the peritoneal cavity.

DESTRUCTIVE OPERATIONS
ON THE FETUS

Most conditions will be most safely managed by Caesarean section despite the fetus being dead or unviable. A destructive operation may be planned before the onset of labour to allow vaginal delivery of an unviable hydrocephalic fetus or it may be carried out in obstructed labour with a dead fetus in a situation where Caesarean section is not a viable option, e.g. when the patient refuses surgery in a developed country or in a third world scenario.

1 **For delivery of an unviable hydrocephalic fetus**
- The prognosis and the procedure to be carried out must be fully discussed before the onset of labour with the mother and her partner.
- Adequate and appropriate analgesia and sedation should be given.
- If cephalic presentation, the head needs to be decompressed to allow its passage through the birth canal.
- In a case of gross hydrocephalus this may be achieved by the release of the cerebrospinal fluid using a spinal needle. This may allow delivery of the fetus but the fetus may well be born alive.
- If breech presentation, when there is a coexisting spina bifida, a catheter or Drew Smyth cannula can be passed up the spinal canal and into the brain to drain the fluid.
- If there is no spina bifida the head can be decompressed trans-abdominally under ultrasound control or vaginally through the foramen magnum.

2 **For obstructed labour with a dead fetus in a situation where Caesarean section is not a viable option**

Craniotomy
This is indicated when there has been a neglected labour and the head is impacted and labour is obstructed.
(a) Direct crushing of the head using the cranioclast or cephalotribe is obsolete.
(b) Catheterize the patient.
(c) Disempact the head from behind the symphysis pubis to allow its passage and to completely empty the bladder.
(d) Make an incision in the posterior part of the fetal scalp and insert the index finger of the left hand under the skin to trace the suture line posteriorly to the fontanelle.
(e) Guide scissors by the finger through the fontanelle into the skull and then open to make a cruciate opening.
(f) Evacuate the brain tissue digitally.
(g) Then attach Kocher's forceps to the lips of incision.
(h) A weight is attached to the forceps and delivery can be expected to take place within a few hours.

(i) This procedure does not depend on the cervix being fully dilated.

(j) Postoperatively the bladder should be drained and antibiotics given.

Decapitation

This is indicated for a shoulder presentation with a dead fetus

(a) In a case of shoulder presentation with obstructed labour and a dead fetus there is a serious risk of uterine rupture.

(b) If decapitation is carried out there is a grave risk of damage to the lower segment.

(c) An arm should be brought down if possible and if the fetus is macerated the fetus may be delivered by traction.

(d) A small fetus may be decapitated using scissors.

(e) A larger or less accessible fetus will require a Blond–Heidler saw, the saw is threaded around the fetal neck. Avoid damage to the vagina by keeping the handles of the saw close together.

(f) The body is delivered by traction on the arm.

(g) The stump of the neck is manipulated and grasped by Volsellum forceps and a finger placed in the mouth to flex the head to deliver it as the after-coming head of a breech.

(h) If gross disproportion is present it will be safer to carry out a Caesarean section.

3 **For shoulder impaction with a dead or non-viable fetus, e.g. a large anencephalic fetus**

Cleidotomy (division of the clavicles)

(a) It is carried out with strong scissors.

(b) If carried out on a live fetus the subclavian artery is likely to be damaged.

CONSULT OTHER TOPICS

Abnormal presentations and positions (p. 34)
Cord prolapse (p. 61)
Postpartum genital tract trauma (p. 104)
Puerperal sepsis, septicaemia and septic shock (p. 113)
Risk management (p. 185)
Shoulder dystocia (p. 119)
Uterine rupture (p. 125)

SUPPLEMENTARY INFORMATION

For obstructed labour with a dead fetus in a situation where Caesarean section is not a viable option

Likely causes of fetal death

- Placental failure due to postmaturity or prolonged labour.
- Excessive moulding of the cephalically presenting fetal head or trapping of the unmoulded head of a breech by an undilated cervix which may fail to descend because of fetopelvic disproportion.

Destructive Operations on the Fetus

- Prolapse of the cord in shoulder or compound presentation.
- Severe intrauterine infection.
- Rupture of the uterus.

REFERENCE

Giwa-Osagie OF and Azzan BB (1987) Destructive operations. *Progress in Obstetrics and Gynaecology*, Vol. 6, pp. 211–221.

ECLAMPSIA, PRE-ECLAMPSIA, HELLP, FATTY LIVER AND HEPATIC RUPTURE

E. O'Donnell, K. Grady and C. Cox

The Report on Confidential Enquiries into Maternal Deaths 1994–1996 found pregnancy induced hypertension as the second leading cause of direct deaths and to have caused 20 deaths. Two deaths were due to fatty liver of pregnancy.

- **Eclampsia** is fitting associated with the syndrome of pre-eclampsia. Seizures can however, occur without any premonitory signs or symptoms.
- **Pre-eclampsia** is pregnancy induced hypertension in association with proteinuria of > 0.5 g/24 hours. It is a multisystem rather than a primary hypertensive disorder.
- **HELLP** is a syndrome comprising haemolysis, elevated liver enzymes and low platelets. It commonly occurs in pre-eclamptic patients.
- **Fatty liver** presents as non-specific malaise, pain in the epigastrium or right upper quadrant or with more specific liver symptoms, e.g. jaundice or bleeding. It can progress to liver failure and rupture. Its symptoms and signs overlap with HELLP syndrome.
- **Hepatic rupture** – the deposition of fibrin-like material in the hepatic sinusoids causes right upper quadrant or epigastric pain which can progress to intrahepatic haemorrhage, subcapsular haematoma and hepatic rupture.

ACTION PLAN

1 **Call for help including senior obstetrician and anaesthetist and inform consultant obstetrician and consultant anaesthetist**

2 **Consider capability of resources and environment for dealing with mother and baby**

3 **Treat and prevent fits**

4 **Deliver the baby or continuously monitor FH by cardiotocography**

5 **Treat hypertension and effect plasma volume expansion**

6 **Pay meticulous attention to fluid balance**

7 **Monitor for and treat complications**

8 **Review maternal and fetal condition regularly**

9 **Document condition of patient, treatment and treatment plan in the notes with time, date, a signature and printed identification**

CONSULT OTHER TOPICS

Airway obstruction (p. 1)
Cardiopulmonary resuscitation (p. 8)

Hypertension (p. 147)
Intrauterine death (p. 81)
Loss of consciousness or fitting (p. 157)
Magnesium toxicity (p. 160)
Massive obstetric haemorrhage – antepartum (p. 88)
Massive obstetric haemorrhage – DIC (p. 92)
Neonatal resuscitation (p. 14)
Oliguria and anuria (p. 162)
Peri-arrest arrhythmias (p. 16)
Premature labour (p. 110)
Respiratory emergencies (p. 20)

SUPPLEMENTARY INFORMATION

Consider capability of resources and environment for dealing with mother and baby

Communicate with a specialist centre in complex cases.

High dependency care is required, to include a resident senior obstetrician and anaesthetist, the availability of invasive monitoring and intensive care and a one-to-one midwife to patient ratio. The condition and needs of the baby might require an *in utero* transfer but this should only be undertaken if the mother is in a stable condition and the resources and personnel are available to transfer her safely.

Treat in high risk area of labour ward and monitor pulse, NIBP, CVP/PCWP, SaO_2, RR, neurological status and reflexes, fluid balance and urine output and FH.

Treat and prevent fits

Assume fit to be eclamptic until proved otherwise. 44% of seizures are post-partum, 38% antepartum and 18% intrapartum.

Airway

- Assess.
- Maintain patency.
- Apply oxygen 15 l/min via tight fitting face mask with reservoir bag.
- Attach pulse oximeter to patient.
- Consider tracheal intubation.

Breathing

- Assess.
- Ventilate.
- Protect airway.

Circulation

- Assess pulse and BP.
- CPR.
- Tilt to left.
- Put on ECG and automatic BP monitor.
- Treat peri-arrest arrhythmias.
- Secure i.v. access with large bore cannula, send bloods for FBC (including

platelets), U&Es, LFTs, uric acid levels, coagulation screen and cross-match 2 units.
- Start i.v. normal saline infusion *slowly*.

Give magnesium sulphate to treat, prevent or prevent recurrent fit

Magnesium sulphate appears to be substantially more effective than phenytoin or diazepam for the treatment of eclampsia.

- This regimen is used for prophylaxis and for treatment of a fit.
- Give a loading dose of 4 g over 5–10 min, followed by a continuous infusion of 1 g/hour (5 g in 200 ml of normal saline over 4 hours). Recurrent seizures should be treated by a further bolus of 2 g.
- If repeated seizures occur despite magnesium, options include diazepam 10 mg i.v. or thiopentone, intubation and ventilation.
- Magnesium infusion should be continued for 24 hours provided tendon reflexes are present and urine output more than 30 ml/hour. If urine output is normal, serum magnesium levels do not need to be measured. If the urine output falls (to less than 100 ml in 4 hours) serum magnesium levels should be measured (therapeutic plasma level 2–4 mmol/l) and close attention paid to signs of developing toxicity.
- If the patient is hyperreflexic and/or has clonus at the ankle or knee or develops other signs of impending eclampsia such as confusion, jitteriness or severe headache, prophylactic magnesium sulphate should be commenced.
- Phenytoin or nimodipine may be used but should be discussed with senior medical staff.
- Carry out a CT scan if fitting has been persistent or if there are neurological signs. Move patient to CT room only when anaesthetist is present and satisfied with airway, ventilation and haemodynamic status.
- In the postpartum period, if thought to be at high risk of fitting, continue anticonvulsants for as long as the patient is hyperreflexic.
- Patient should remain in labour ward for at least 24 hours after the last fit.

Deliver the baby or continuously monitor FH by cardiotocography

Although delivery is the definitive treatment, the mother must be stabilized first of all. If baby is dead consider induction of labour. If baby alive in selected patients labour may be induced. The following must apply to proceed to vaginal delivery:

- stable maternal condition
- no fetal distress
- cephalic presentation
- favourable cervix and, if eclamptic, no further fits

Treat hypertension and effect plasma volume expansion

Antihypertensive treatment benefits the mother with mild (diastolic 90–99 mmHg) to moderate (diastolic 100–109 mmHg) hypertension but there is no clear choice of drugs. For severe hypertension (diastolic > 110 mmHg), morbidity and mortality related to prematurity are significant in women with acute severe hypertension before 34 weeks' gestation, if they are stabilized and delivered. Therefore, a more expectant approach has been advocated where the average prolongation of pregnancy was 2 weeks.

Severe hypertension should be treated in an area with invasive monitoring facilities. Regular NIBP and ECG monitoring is necessary and consider intra-arterial blood pressure monitoring if BP unstable.

The choice of antihypertensive should depend on the experience and familiarity of an individual clinician with a particular drug.

Nifedipine 10 mg orally or sublingually (with 300 ml of synthetic colloid to avoid precipitous fall in BP – if preicipitous fall in BP occurs ephedrine in 3 mg increments should be given i.v. and titrated against BP) is suggested and can be repeated every 30 min according to response. Maintenance can be given as a slow release preparation 10 mg BD increasing to 20 mg BD. An interaction between nifedipine and magnesium sulphate has been reported to produce profound maternal muscle weakness, maternal hypotension and fetal distress. The risk is small but labetolol may be preferred if magnesium sulphate is being used.

Labetolol is given as an initial i.v. bolus of 5 mg titrated against blood pressure and repeated at 5 min intervals up to a dose of 1 mg/kg. Labetolol can precipitate heart failure and its use must be closely observed.

Hydralazine is commonly used. If there is no great urgency, the mother should receive a pre-loading infusion of 400 ml of 4.5% human albumin given over 20 minutes. Give 5 mg i.v. slowly. The onset of antihypertensive effect may be delayed. Additional doses can be given to a maximum dose of 20 mg, but only at intervals of 20 minutes. The effect of a single dose may last up to 6 hours. If no lasting effect with boluses (assess over 20 min), consider an infusion at 2.0 mg/hour increasing by 0.5 mg/hour as required (2–20 mg/hour usually required).

It has been found that, compared with intravenous hydralazine, nifedipine and labetolol were associated with less maternal hypotension, fewer Caesarean sections, fewer placental abruptions and fewer low Apgar scores.

If blood pressure does not respond to the above discuss with senior renal physicians and senior anaesthetists who will supervise further treatment.

Epidural analgesia can be used to control blood pressure. It is only indicated if the patient is in labour and is contraindicated in the presence of a coagulopathy.

Plasma volume expansion is necessary because in severe pre-eclampsia there is an increase in systemic vascular resistance. If this is reduced by anti-hypertensives, a precipitous fall in blood pressure can result. The ideal is to gently reduce the systemic vascular resistance and simultaneously expand the intravascular volume, thereby improving end organ blood flow.

Postpartum, continue antihypertensives if diastolic > 110 mmHg or mean arterial pressure > 140 mmHg.

Pay meticulous attention to fluid balance

- Patient is in net fluid overload, but the fluid has leaked out of the intravascular compartment due to low oncotic pressure and increased capillary permeability.

  Do not put patient at risk through iatrogenic overload. No woman with severe pre-eclampsia/eclampsia should have a net crystalloid intake of > 2.5 l/24 hours as maintenance.
- Insert indwelling urinary catheter and keep strict intake/output charts with running totals. Give the previous hour's urinary output plus 40–50 ml (beware chasing the natural diuresis that occurs postdelivery; only rarely should the total maintenance be more than 2.5 l). The fluid used should be guided by the electrolytes. (Beware hyponatraemia < 135 mmol/l.) Check U&Es every 8 hours.
- If the average urine output is less than 25 ml/hour over 4 hours, this is usually due to decreased intravascular volume and will respond to 200 ml of synthetic colloid which can be repeated if necessary.

- Be guided by CVP which should measure 0–5 cmH$_2$O. It can be misleading, however, as a low CVP (filling pressure for the right side of the heart) can be found in the presence of a high pulmonary capillary wedge pressure (filling pressure for the left side of the heart). In the presence of pre-eclampsia and haemorrhage, a falling CVP trend is a useful guide. If oliguria persists consult senior anaesthetists and renal team to consider other options such as pulmonary artery catheter measurements and low dose dopamine infusion.
- In the presence of over-hydration, particularly with heart failure or impending renal failure, frusemide/furosemide 10–20 mg i.v. should be considered.
- Check urinary electrolytes and osmolarity only if early renal failure is suspected
- If syntocinon is needed, in order to reduce the total fluid input prepare 4 units of syntocinon in 50 ml in an infusion. Start at 1.5 ml/hour, doubling the rate every 30 min to a maximum of 18 ml/hour. Do not give ergometrine or syntometrine.

Monitor for and treat complications

Warning features are:

- headache, visual disturbances, epigastric pain, vomiting,
- peripheral (especially facial) or pulmonary oedema,
- RUQ tenderness,
- optic vasospasm,
- recently developed hypertension > 160/110 with proteinuria > 1 g/24 hours,
- Hyperreflexia and rapidly changing biochemical/haematological picture.

Respiratory complications

These occur from pulmonary oedema, over-sedation and aspiration, and laryngeal oedema causing respiratory obstruction. Oxygen saturation should be > 95% and additional humidified oxygen given by face mask or nasal cannulae. If oxygen saturation is not > 95% without oxygen there is a problem.

Arrange CXR if oxygen saturation not > 95% or if RR > 25 beats/min or if aspiration suspected.

Cardiac complications

Beware of over-hydration, arrhythmias.

Renal complications

Renal failure may develop secondary to hypertension or hypovolaemia or as a primary injury in severe pre-eclampsia.

Neurological complications

Cerebral oedema is a life-threatening complication.

Baseline examination is pupillary and tendon reflexes and Glasgow Coma Score.

Haematological complications

Check haemoglobin, platelets and coagulation screen every 8 hours. It is not necessary to routinely check fibrinogen levels and FDPs.

If the platelet count is in excess of $100 \times 10^9/l$ a coagulation problem is unlikely. Spontaneous haemorrhage may occur if platelets less than $40 \times 10^9/l$. If so give platelets. If frank DIC give fresh frozen plasma. Consider cryo-precipitate if fibrinogen levels are < 100 units.

Retinal complications

Always do fundoscopy at the time of review (unless impending eclampsia) to exclude arterial and venous haemorrhages, papilloedema and retinal detachment.

Hepatic complications

Daily LFTs are necessary. Deposits of fibrin-like material in the hepatic sinusoids cause elevation of the liver enzymes (sometimes only minimal).

Fatty liver may cause hypoglycaemia, coagulopathy, encephalopathy, liver rupture and multiple organ failure. Is associated with significant maternal mortality and requires intensive supportive therapy.

The patient with spontaneous rupture of the liver presents with persistent pain after delivery. Alternatively acute hypotension may be the only symptom. Diagnosis is made by CT scan. If the patient is stable with no evidence of free intra-abdominal fluid, manage conservatively with aggressive blood product replacement. If acute hypotension perform immediate laparotomy. The more usual treatment at laparotomy is evacuation of haematoma and packing. Lobectomy has also been used. If the patient requires a second packing due to persistent major bleeding from the liver, selective embolization during hepatic angiography may be used.

Fetal complications

These include intrauterine growth retardation, fetal distress in labour, preterm delivery and intrauterine death due to placental abruption or asphyxia in labour. Umbilical artery Doppler wave form is a strong and independent predictor of adverse perinatal outcome and should be undertaken where possible.

Review maternal and fetal condition regularly

The patient should, at a minimum be reviewed by a consultant obstetrician daily and by the SpR/SHO every 4 hours.

Review pulse, NIBP, CVP/PCWP, SaO_2, RR, neurological status and reflexes, fluid balance and urine output and FH.

The following should be recorded by the SpR/SHO every 4 hours.

(a) Change in symptoms; beware confusion and persistent visual disturbance.
(b) Full chest examination, looking particularly for early pulmonary oedema.
(c) Level of consciousness (Glasgow Coma Scale [GCS]), reflexes (particularly clonus) and fundoscopy.
(d) Running total of intake and output over previous 4 hours and previous 24 hours.
(e) Total dose of antihypertensive and anticonvulsant drug used.

SYSTEMATIC REVIEWS

Duley L and Henderson-Smart D (1999) Magnesium sulphate versus phenytoin for eclampsia (Cochrane Review). *The Cochrane Library*, Issue 2. Update Software, Oxford.

Reviewers' conclusions: *Magnesium sulphate appears to be substantially more effective than phenytoin for the treatment of eclampsia.*

Duley L and Henderson-Smart D (1999) Magnesium sulphate versus diazepam for eclampsia (Cochrane review). *The Cochrane Library*, Issue 2. Update Software, Oxford.

Reviewers' conclusions: *Magnesium sulphate appears to be substantially more effective than diazepam for the treatment of eclampsia.*

Duley L, Gulmezoglu AM and Henderson-Smart DJ (1999) Anticonvulsants for pre-eclampsia (Cochrane Review). *The Cochrane Library*, Issue 2. Update Software, Oxford.

Reviewers' conclusions: *There is not enough evidence to establish the benefits and hazards of anticonvulsants for pre-eclampsia. If an anticonvulsant is used, magnesium sulphate appears to be the best choice.*

Duley L and Henderson-Smart DJ (1999) Drugs for rapid treatment of very high blood pressure during pregnancy (Cochrane Review). *The Cochrane Library*, Issue 2. Update Software, Oxford.

Reviewers' conclusions: *Until better evidence is available, the choice of antihypertensive should depend on the experience and familiarity of an individual clinician with a particular drug, and on what is known about adverse maternal and fetal side-effects. Exceptions are diazoxide and ketanserin, which are probably not good choices.*

Hofmeyr GJ (1999) Abdominal decompression for suspected fetal compromise/pre-eclampsia (Cochrane Review). *The Cochrane Library*, Issue 2. Update Software, Oxford.

Reviewers' conclusions: *Due to the methodological limitations of the studies, the effects of therapeutic abdominal decompression are not clear. The apparent improvements in birth weight and perinatal mortality warrant further evaluation of abdominal decompression where there is impaired fetal growth and possibly for women with pre-eclampsia.*

Offringa M (1998) Excess mortality after human albumin administration in critically ill patients. *Clinical and pathophysiological evidence suggests albumin is harmful.* Br. Med. J. **317**: 223–224.

REFERENCES

Eclampsia Trial Collaborative Group (1995) Which anticonvulsant for women with eclampsia? *Lancet* **345**: 1455–1463.

Magee LA, Ornstein MP and von Dadelzen P (1999) Management of hypertension in pregnancy. *Br. Med. J.* **318**: 1299–1362.

RCOG (1996) *Guidelines on the Management of Eclampsia*. Royal College of Obstetricians and Gynaecologists, London.

FEMALE GENITAL MUTILATION (CIRCUMCISION) – COMPLICATIONS

M.A. Khaled, M.E.F. Saad and C. Cox

This is the practice of excision, infibulation or other mutilation of the whole or any part of the labia majora or clitoris of another person. The definition of infibulation is 'a stitching together of the labia'.

When an obstetrician is faced with the repair of the vulva of a woman who has delivered a baby vaginally following a previous infibulation, surgery can be performed for purposes connected with the labour and the birth, but it is illegal to repair the labia intentionally in such a way that intercourse is difficult or impossible – Prohibition of Female Circumcision Act 1985.

To reverse infibulation

The patient should be assessed preconceptually and the infibulation reversed before the first pregnancy if possible. If discovered during pregnancy, the infibulation should be reversed during the midtrimester. It may be necessary to deal with the infibulation at the time of delivery.

ACTION PLAN

1 **Prior to labour, under anaesthesia, examine the vulva and insert a probe under the scar**

2 **Open the scar in the midline revealing the underlying tissues which may include an intact hymen**

3 **Carry the incision forward to expose the clitoral area**

4 **Consider potential complications in pregnancy and delivery**

5 **During labour incision of the infibulation scar should be carried out as the head distends the perineum**

6 **Document findings and procedures in notes with time, date, a signature and printed identification**

CONSULT OTHER TOPICS

Instrumental delivery – forceps (p. 75)
Instrumental delivery – ventouse (p. 78)
Massive obstetric haemorrhage – antepartum (p. 88)
Massive obstetric haemorrhage – DIC (p. 92)
Massive obstetric haemorrhage – postpartum (p. 95)
Postpartum genital tract trauma (p. 104)
Risk management (p. 185)

SUPPLEMENTARY INFORMATION

Consider potential complications in pregnancy and delivery

Antenatally

Difficulty in diagnosing urinary infections – pus cells in the urine do not necessarily indicate a urinary tract infection as the urine is frequently contaminated by vaginal secretions which collect under the infibulation scar. A vulval wash followed by a midstream collection is advisable.

Infection of epidermoid inclusion cysts (a not uncommon complication) should be managed by incision or excision under adequate analgesia or anaesthesia.

First stage of labour

Narrowing of the introitus leads to difficulty in assessing the progress of labour; rectal examination may be helpful to establish progressive cervical dilatation and to aid the decision with regard to incising the infibulation scar.

Psychological distress and apprehension is likely and adequate analgesia for labour and any procedures on the vulva is essential. An epidural anaesthetic is ideal.

Second stage of labour

Presence of a bulky epidermoid vulval inclusion cyst: even if bulky this should be left undisturbed as it is quite possible to incise the infibulation scar in the midline after pushing the cyst to one side. Inclusion cysts should be dealt with as an elective procedure after the puerperium.

Delay in the second stage: the presence of the scar is not an indication for or a contraindication to an instrumental delivery.

Bleeding from vulval and vaginal lacerations may result from extensions to the incision or from uncontrolled rupture of the scar. These lacerations will normally be repaired after the delivery of the placenta. More major bleeding from arterial spurters can be controlled by the use of haemostatic forceps. These lacerations may involve the inner aspects of the labia majora and can extend to involve the suburethral area. A catheter will be advisable in cases of spiral suburethral tears. A low threshhold for an episiotomy should be employed.

Third stage of labour

Postpartum haemorrhage from lacerations may be severe and requires adequate analgesia to facilitate examination and repair.

Puerperium

Urinary retention is more common after suburethral lacerations; a catheter should be passed and antibiotic cover considered.

Vulval or vaginal haematomas should be managed in the normal way.

Infection of wound or retention cysts may require drainage under regional or general anaesthesia.

Psychological support should be available as necessary.

REFERENCE

(1992) Female Circumcision (female genital mutilation). *Int. J. Gynaecol. and Obstet.* **37**: 149.

Female Genital Mutilation (Circumcision) – Complications

INSTRUMENTAL DELIVERY – FORCEPS

Richard Johanson and Charles Cox

The Royal College of Obstetricians and Gynaecologists' Audit Standard states that 'the Ventouse should be the instrument of first choice for operative vaginal delivery'. It is important, however, that the operator uses an instrument, either forceps or ventouse, with which he/she is experienced.

ACTION PLAN

1 **Consider indications for instrumental delivery**

2 **Ensure criteria for forceps delivery**

3 **Palpate abdomen to confirm head is fully engaged**
- Abdominal palpation must be carried out particularly in cases of face presentation.

4 **Provide analgesia**

5 **Catheterize the bladder**

6 **Perform vaginal examination to confirm the cervix is fully dilated and check the position of the head**

7 **Select appropriate forceps**

8 **Check the forceps blades fit together before and after application**

9 **Apply blades and pull with contractions**
- A maximum of three pulls. Pull downwards at 45 degrees.

10 **Episiotomy is usually required**

11 **Repair episiotomy and carry out rectal examination to check sphincter and rectal mucosa for tears**

12 **Check swabs and instruments**

13 **Document the indications and procedure fully with date, time, a signature and printed identification**

CONSULT OTHER TOPICS

SUPPLEMENTARY INFORMATION

Consider indications for instrumental delivery

- Prolonged second stage. There is no absolute limit or correct length for the second stage but certain situations may warrant a non-pushing second stage or shortened second stage.
- Cardiorespiratory compromise.
- Retinal detachment.
- Eclampsia and severe pre-eclampsia.
- Intrapartum haemorrhage.
- Cord prolapse.
- Dural tap.
- Second twin.
- After prolonged pushing when the risk of fetal hypoxia increases as does the risk of postpartum haemorrhage.

Specific indication:

- Fetuses at increased risk of fetal distress such as prematurity or intrauterine growth retardation.

Ensure criteria for forceps delivery

- Full engagement of the head.
- Full dilation of the cervix.

Provide analgesia

- For mid-cavity forceps, epidural top-up or spinal are preferred, but pudendal nerve block and local anaesthetic infiltration are an option.
- For rotational forceps, general anaesthetic, spinal or epidural analegesia is necessary.

Select appropriate forceps

Rotational forceps delivery should only be carried out by people trained in the technique. In the occipito-posterior position, blades may be applied directly with the operator hand between the fetal head and the vaginal wall. For the occipito-transverse position, the posterior blade is applied directly and the anterior blade is inserted between the baby's face and the operator's hand and 'wandered' over the face to the parietal region anteriorly. Rotation is achieved between contractions and after rotation has been achieved the baby can either be delivered with a Kielland's forceps or some operators prefer to remove the Kielland's and deliver the baby with midcavity forceps to reduce damage to the maternal perineum. Rotational forceps should not be used without adequate analgesia.

Forceps may also be used at Caesarean section to assist delivery of the head.

Mid-cavity or low cavity (Wrigley's) forceps may be used to protect the fetal head in premature delivery.

Mid-cavity forceps may be used to deliver the after-coming head of a breech.

SYSTEMATIC REVIEWS

Johanson RB and Menon BKV (1999) Vacuum extraction versus forceps for assisted vaginal delivery (Cochrane Review). *The Cochrane Library*, Issue 2. Update Software, Oxford.

Reviewers' conclusions: *Use of the vacuum extractor rather than forceps for assisted delivery appears to reduce maternal morbidity. The reduction in cephalhaematoma and retinal haemorrhages seen with forceps may be a compensatory benefit.*

Johanson R and Menon V (1999) Soft versus rigid vacuum extractor cups for assisted vaginal delivery (Cochrane Review). *The Cochrane Library*, Issue 2. Update Software, Oxford.

Reviewers' conclusions: *Metal cups appear to be more suitable for 'occipito-posterior', transverse and difficult 'occipito-anterior' position deliveries. The soft cups seem to be appropriate for straightforward deliveries.*

INSTRUMENTAL DELIVERY – VENTOUSE

Richard Johanson and Charles Cox

The Royal College of Obstetricians and Gynaecologists' Audit Standard states that 'the Ventouse should be the instrument of first choice for operative vaginal delivery'. It is important however that the operator uses an instrument, either forceps or ventouse with which he/she is familiar, comfortable and experienced.

1 **Consider indications for instrumental delivery**

2 **Ensure criteria for ventouse delivery**

3 **Palpate abdomen to confirm head is engaged** and to assess size of the baby

4 **Perform vaginal examination**
- To confirm that the fetal head is engaged and that the cervix is fully dilated.
- Also to assess the position and attitude of the baby's head (flexed/deflexed) and the adequacy of the maternal pelvis.
- An assessment of the amount of caput and moulding should be made.

5 **Provide perineal analgesia**

6 **It may be necessary to catheterize the bladder. This must be done if the patient has an epidural**

7 **Select the appropriate cup**
- The silicone rubber cup is used with well flexed cephalic presentations.
- The anterior metal cup is used for large babies, if the second stage is prolonged and if there is a moderate degree of caput.
- The posterior metal cup is used for deflexed posterior positions.

8 **Apply the cup as near to the occiput as possible**
- Take the pressure up to 0.2 kg/cm^2.
- Check no maternal tissue is caught under the cup then up to 0.8 kg/cm^2.

9 **Begin traction with the next contraction**
- The direction of pull is downwards at an angle of 45° from the horizontal.

10 **Rest one hand on the bell of the cup while the other applies traction**

11 **Use operator fingers on the head to promote flexion and guide the head under the arch of the pubis. When head crowns change the angle of traction through an arc of 90° upwards.**

12 **An episiotomy is cut if required but may not be necessary, e.g. in a multiparous patient with fetal distress**

13 **Repair episiotomy and carry out rectal examination to check the sphincter and rectal mucosa for tears**

14 **If ventouse fails consider reasons**

15 **Check swabs and instruments**

16 **Document the indications and procedure fully with date, time, a signature and printed identification**

CONSULT OTHER TOPICS

SUPPLEMENTARY INFORMATION

Consider indications for instrumental delivery

- Prolonged second stage. There is no absolute limit or correct length for the second stage but certain situations may warrant a non-pushing second stage or shortened second stage.
- Cardiorespiratory compromise.
- Retinal detachment.
- Eclampsia and severe pre-eclampsia.
- Intrapartum haemorrhage.
- Cord prolapse.
- Dural tap.
- Second twin.
- After prolonged pushing when the risk of fetal hypoxia increases as does the risk of postpartum haemorrhage.

Specific indication:

- Fetuses at increased risk of fetal distress such as prematurity or intrauterine growth retardation.

Ensure criteria for ventouse delivery

- Full engagement of the head.
- Full dilatation of cervix.
- A cooperative patient.
- The presence of good contractions.
- The delivery should be completed within 15 min of the application.

- The head should descend with each pull.
- The cup should be reapplied no more than twice.

Palpate abdomen to to confirm that the head is engaged

None of the head should be palpable abdominally.

Provide perineal analgesia

If there is an existing epidural, this can be topped up. It is usually only necessary to infiltrate with local anaesthetic.

If ventouse fails consider reasons

- Misdiagnosis of engagement or position.
- Using the wrong cup.
- Inadequate assessment of the pelvis and position of the baby's head.
- Incorrect placement of the cup .
- Wrong angle of traction.
- Excessive caput .
- Poor maternal effort.
- True cephalopelvic disproportion.

If failure with the ventouse occurs despite good traction DO NOT apply the forceps.

SYSTEMATIC REVIEWS

Johanson RB and Menon BKV (1999) Vacuum extraction versus forceps for assisted vaginal delivery (Cochrane Review). *The Cochrane Library*, Issue 2. Update Software, Oxford.

Reviewers' conclusions: *Use of the vacuum extractor rather than forceps for assisted delivery appears to reduce maternal morbidity. The reduction in cephalhaematoma and retinal haemorrhages seen with forceps may be a compensatory benefit.*

Johanson RB and Menon BKV (1999) Soft versus rigid vacuum extractor cups for assisted vaginal delivery (Cochrane Review). *The Cochrane Library*, Issue 2. Update Software, Oxford.

Reviewers' conclusions: *Metal cups appear to be more suitable for 'occipito-posterior', transverse and difficult 'occipito-anterior' position deliveries. The soft cups seem to be appropriate for straightforward deliveries.*

INTRAUTERINE DEATH

E. O'Donnell and C. Cox

Intrauterine death is diagnosed by the absence of fetal heart activity confirmed by an experienced ultrasonographer.

1 **Inform patient in the presence of witnesses, preferably her partner or other friend or relation**

2 **A cause of death should be sought**

3 **A vaginal delivery should be planned unless there are contraindications or relative contraindications**

4 **Investigations should follow a protocol which may vary from hospital to hospital**

5 **Consider timing of delivery**
- Immediate delivery is rarely indicated and timing of the delivery should be based on the patient's wishes but imminent delivery is indicated in the presence of haemorrhage, suspected placental abruption, sepsis, coagulopathy or ruptured membranes.

6 **Manage labour as follows**
- Prime uterus with mifipristone 200 mg 36 hours before cervagem to facilitate induction.
- Induce with cervagem.
- The membranes are ruptured only when labour is well established because of the risk of infection.
- Adequate analgesia should be offered, usually an epidural (unless there is a coagulation disorder).
- Labour should be augmented as normally indicated.
- Instrumental delivery and episiotomy should be avoided if possible.
- A broad spectrum antibiotic should be considered.
- Continuity of caregiver should be provided wherever possible.

7 **Attend to mother and father's needs**

8 **Further investigate the cause of intrauterine death**

9 **Be aware of potential complications**

10 **Attend to issues of risk management**

11 **Issue a certificate of still birth and ensure that mother realizes that the birth must be registered with the Registrar of Births and Deaths within 42 days of delivery**

CONSULT OTHER TOPICS

Destructive operations on the fetus (p. 63)
Puerperal sepsis, septicaemia and septic shock (p. 113)
Risk management (p. 185)

SUPPLEMENTARY INFORMATION

Inform patient in the presence of witnesses, preferably her partner or other friend or relation

Allow them time to digest the information and to have ultrasonography repeated on another occasion if necessary, as there is no evidence that speedy termination of the pregnancy reduces distress.

A vaginal delivery should be planned unless there are contraindications or relative contraindications, such as

- Placenta praevia.
- Multiple previous Caesarean sections, a classical Caesarean section or an operation involving opening the cavity of the uterus such as a myomectomy.
- Suspected rupture of the uterus.
- Obstructed labour where a destructive operation would be necessary to effect vaginal delivery, e.g. severe cephalopelvic disproportion, impacted transverse lie or shoulder presentation.

Investigations should follow a protocol which may vary from hospital to hospital

This will usually include the following.

- Full blood count including platelets and a clotting screen if the fetus has been dead for more than 2 weeks.
- Kleihauer test, blood group and check antibodies.
- Urea and electrolytes, liver function tests.
- TORCH screen, parvovirus antibodies and listeria antibodies.
- Random blood sugar and Hb A1 glycosylated haemoglobin.
- Anticardiolipin and autoimmune antibody screen.

Consider timing of delivery

- With conservative management 80% will deliver within 2 weeks but the majority opt for an induced delivery.
- If delivery is delayed, monitoring for infection and coagulopathy is mandatory. Coagulopathy rarely occurs at less than 20 weeks' gestation or if the fetus has been dead less than 4 weeks.
- Swabs should be taken from the vagina and cervix to identify chlamydia and other organisms such as B-haemolytic streptococcus. Sepsis is rare as long as the membranes remain intact.

Attend to the mother and father's needs

- Photographs should be taken as soon as possible with a polaroid camera so that there is an immediate record for the mother. Other professional photos should be taken by the medical illustration department later.

- The mother and partner should be encouraged to look at and hold the baby.
- Momentos of the baby should be preserved, e.g. locks of hair.
- Offer mother suppression of lactation with cabergoline 1 mg within 24 hours of delivery.
- If possible the mother should be offered an individual room where her partner can stay.
- Information about support groups should be given, e.g. SANDS (Stillbirth and Neonatal Death Society).
- Follow up and support services (community and GP services) must be arranged before she leaves hospital.

Further investigate the cause of intrauterine death

- Permission should be requested for a postmortem examination and if refused this should be clearly recorded in the notes.
- Check that the maternal bloods have been sent for the stillbirth screening tests.
- Send placenta for examination (swab for bacteriology, biopsy for karyotype and histology).
- Send fetal blood or tissue for karyotyping and viral studies.
- Consider X-rays, e.g. in dwarfism, or particularly if a postmortem has been refused.
- If the fetus is abnormal consider karyotyping the parents.

Be aware of potential complications

- Infection is more likely as dead material is a good culture medium. The membranes should be kept intact as long as is reasonable.
- Swabs should be taken and an antibiotic given.
- If the fetus has been dead for more than 2 weeks there is a small risk of a coagulopathy. The platelet count should be checked at regular intervals; if there is a drop then a full clotting screen should be done.

Attend to issues of risk management

- Record the sequence of events fully with contemporaneous, legible notes. If information needs to be added in retrospect, this should be clearly recorded, signed and dated.
- The consultant responsible for her care must be informed. If on leave, a written communication should be left with the secretary.
- Recheck that all the appropriate investigations have been done and the protocol complied with fully.
- Ensure general practitioner and community midwife have been informed.
- Check that the mother is in possession of the photographs of the baby.
- Ensure that follow-up appointments have been made.
- Discuss at perinatal morbidity/mortality meeting.

USEFUL TELEPHONE NUMBERS

Stillbirth and Neonatal Death Society (SANDS)	0171 436 5881
CRUSE (Care for the Bereaved)	0181 940 4818
British Association for Counselling	01788 578328

SYSTEMATIC REVIEW

Chambers HM and Chan FY (1999) Support for women/families after perinatal death (Cochrane Review). *The Cochrane Library*, Issue 2. Update Software, Oxford.

Reviewers' conclusions: *No information is available from randomized trials to indicate whether there is or is not a benefit from providing specific psychological support or counselling after perinatal death.*

INVERTED UTERUS

Inversion of the uterus is defined as the passage of the fundus of the uterus through the cervix. Inversion of the uterus can be partial or complete. It does not necessarily imply mismanagement of the third stage.

1 **Suspect**
- If signs of collapse with no obvious bleeding suspect inverted uterus or ruptured uterus.

2 **Airway**
- Assess.
- Maintain patency.
- Apply oxygen 15 l/min via tight fitting face mask with reservoir bag.
- Attach pulse oximeter to patient.
- Call anaesthetist.

Breathing
- Assess.
- Ventilate.
- Protect airway.

Circulation
- Assess pulse and BP.
- CPR.
- Put on ECG and automatic BP monitor.
- Treat peri-arrest arrhythmias.
- i.v. access with large bore cannula, send bloods for FBC and cross-match, start i.v.i.
- The patient may be hypotensive out of proportion to blood loss. This is due to vagal stimulation from the uterus. Be prepared to give atropine 0.6 mg i.v. if bradycardia and consider volume replacement.

3 **Summon senior obstetrician – this is a life-threatening emergency**

4 **Attempt immediate manual replacement of the uterus**

5 **Call anaesthetist if not already present**

6 **Attempt replacement with tocolysis using ritodrine as necessary**
- Ensure adequate analgesia.

7 **Under general anaesthesia attempt to replace uterus**
- Digitally replace that part of the inversion nearest to the cervix first and so on, pushing the uterus high up into the abdomen with the vaginal hand.

8   **If placenta is adherent the inversion should be corrected before attempts are made to separate the placenta**

9   **Consider hydrostatic methods**

10 **If unsuccessful surgical treatment may be required**

11 **Keep record chart of pulse, BP, RR, SaO$_2$ and treatments given**

12 **Record clearly in notes, with time, date, a signature and printed identification and inform consultant obstetrician**

CONSULT OTHER TOPICS

Airway obstruction (p. 1)
Cardiopulmonary resuscitation (p. 8)
Hypotension (p. 150)
Massive obstetric haemorrhage – postpartum (p. 95)
Peri-arrest arrhythmias (p. 16)
Respiratory emergencies (p. 20)
Risk management (p. 185)
Uterine rupture (p. 125)

SUPPLEMENTARY INFORMATION

Suspect

- Continuing PPH despite apparently well contracted uterus.
- Associated lower abdominal pain.
- Dimpled uterine fundus.
- Vaginal mass on examination.
- Shock out of proportion to blood loss.

Attempt immediate manual replacement of the uterus

The sooner it is replaced the better as with time it becomes increasingly difficult to replace the inversion through the contracting cervix.

Consider hydrostatic methods

- O'Sullivans method. Place the nozzle of tubing delivering fluid in the posterior fornix and use the forearm to occlude the vagina. This results in ballooning of the vagina and resolution of the inversion.
- A recent modification uses the Silc ventouse cup to occlude the vagina producing a better seal.

If unsuccessful, surgical treatment may be required

It may help to put traction on the round ligaments to exert traction on the fundus.

- At laparotomy the dimple of the inversion is identified. Allis clamps are used to grasp the uterus below the contraction ring and careful traction is applied. Further clamps are applied as necessary as the inversion is reduced. This is the Huntington procedure.

- If this procedure is unsuccessful a vertical incision should be made posteriorly over the constriction ring, the inversion reduced and the hysterotomy incision repaired. This is the Haultain procedure.

MASSIVE OBSTETRIC HAEMORRHAGE – ANTEPARTUM

The 1994–1996 Report on Confidential Enquiries into Maternal Deaths in the United Kingdom found haemorrhage to be the sixth leading cause of death. Antepartum haemorrhage is bleeding from the genital tract after 24 weeks' gestation. The causes of bleeding before and after 24 weeks are the same.

The incidence is 3% – 1% from placenta praevia, 1% from abruptio placenta and 1% from other causes.

It can be caused by coagulation defects caused by anticoagulant treatment or hereditary conditions such as von Willibrand's disease. Occasionally bleeding may be fetal in the case of vasa praevia.

1 **Suspect**

2 **Call for senior obstetrician, anaesthetist, theatre team, extra midwifery staff and porter to be readily available**

3 **Discuss urgency with haematologist, so that ABO and RhD matched blood can be made available if necessary**

4 **Airway**
- Assess.
- Maintain patency.
- Apply oxygen 15 l/min via tight fitting face mask with reservoir bag.
- Attach pulse oximeter to patient.

Breathing
- Assess.
- Ventilate.
- Protect airway.
- Regularly monitor RR.

Circulation
- CPR if necessary.
- Treat peri-arrest arrhythmias.
- Tilt to left.
- Assess volume loss by overt losses peripheral perfusion, pulse, blood pressure and catheterize and measure urine output half hourly.
- Remember haemorrhage is invariably underestimated.

5 **Replace volume loss**
- Insert two large bore i.v. cannulae.
- Send bloods for FBC, clotting studies, cross-match 6 units and Kleihauer.
- Correct volume loss initially by up to 2 l of normal saline followed by synthetic colloid, then whole blood or packed red cells as soon as they are available.

- If blood loss is life-threatening, group O Rh negative red cells should be used if this is the fastest available source of blood.
- Consider group specific blood, but preferably use fully cross-matched blood.
- Warm i.v. fluids.
- Infuse with a pressure bag.
- Put on automatic NIBP monitor, consider CVP for monitoring and i.v. access, PCWP and arterial pressure monitoring.
- Move to high dependency area of labour ward.

6 **Listen for fetal heart sounds and begin cardiotocography if possible**

7 **Diagnose and treat source of bleeding**

8 **Suspect and aggressively treat coagulopathy in discussion with haematologist**

9 **Check FBC, haematocrit, clotting and arterial blood gases regularly as appropriate**

10 **Consider transfer to HDU/ICU**

11 **Keep a record of pulse, BP, RR, SaO$_2$, CVP, PCWP, urine output, fluids given, laboratory results and FH**

12 **Document in the notes with times, date, a signature and printed identification**

CONSULT OTHER TOPICS

Acute abdominal pain (p. 44)
Airway obstruction (p. 1)
Cardiopulmonary resuscitation (p. 8)
Hypotension (p. 150)
Intrauterine death (p. 81)
Massive obstetric haemorrhage – DIC (p. 92)
Massive obstetric haemorrhage – postpartum (p. 95)
Neonatal resuscitation (p. 14)
Peri-arrest arrhythmias (p. 16)
Respiratory emergencies (p. 20)

SUPPLEMENTARY INFORMATION

Suspect

Bleeding from the placental site

(i) Abruptio placentae ('accidental' haemorrhage)
Bleeding from a normally situated placenta. The bleeding may be concealed or revealed. Sudden onset of severe abdominal pain, shock and tenderness over the uterus with a hard 'woody' feel to the uterus are characteristic symptoms and signs. However, with a posterior placental abruption the abdomen may be soft.

The fetal heart sounds may be muffled or absent. If the baby is dead the abruption is major by definition. Disseminated intravascular coagulation is a common complication. A large placental abruption can occur without any visible vaginal blood loss (concealed haemorrhage).

(ii) Placenta praevia ('inevitable' haemorrhage)
Bleeding from an abnormally situated placenta. Painless bleeding often with no precipitating factor. Fetal heart sounds are usually present and easily heard. Bleeding may be very heavy and will be bright red.

Bleeding from the uterus

Vaginal bleeding may occur from rupture of the uterus either before or after the onset of labour.

A lower segment Caesarean section scar may rupture during labour, characteristically there is pain and tenderness over the lower segment scar with a loss of blood vaginally and cessation of uterine contractions. Fetal heart rate abnormalities are likely to be present.

Unusually the uterus may rupture during pregnancy – this can occur in women who have undergone a classical Caesarean section or women who have had surgery involving the cavity of the uterus, e.g. myomectomy. This will cause pain and usually some vaginal bleeding.

Bleeding from the cervix

Fairly common in pregnancy due to the increased vascularity and ectropion formation on the cervix. Cervical polyps are not uncommon and are more friable in pregnancy. Bleeding is often precipitated by trauma, e.g. intercourse.
Beware carcinoma of the cervix!
The cervix may lacerate and bleed during dilatation in the first stage of labour, particularly if surgery has been performed such as a cone biopsy, Manchester repair or even a large loop excision of the transformation zone (LLETZ).

Bleeding from the vagina or vulva

Bleeding from the vagina is uncommon but may result from local trauma or infection such as candida and the human papilloma virus.

Vulval bleeding may be due to rupture of vulval varices and can be very profuse. It is controlled by direct pressure initially.

Circulation

Ensure adequate transfusion – the best resuscitation for the fetus *in utero* is to resuscitate the mother. Inadequate transfusion is frequent, especially in cases of placental abruption.

Listen for fetal heart sounds and begin cardiotocography if possible

- If significant haemorrhage has occurred and the fetus is viable consider immediate delivery.
- Ultrasound is helpful to confirm if the fetus is alive and to locate the placenta.
- Placenta praevia is more accurately diagnosed by transvaginal scanning.
- If the placenta is normally sited a speculum examination should be carried out to exclude local cervical pathology.
- Vaginal examination should not be carried out until maternal records have been examined and an ultrasound carried out if necessary.

Diagnose and treat source of bleeding

- If Caesarean section is to be carried out for a major abruption or placenta praevia, senior members of staff should be present both from the obstetric and anaesthetic team.
- Induction of labour may be carried out if the fetus is dead. Particular attention should be paid to adequacy of resuscitation and a central line is likely to be of value. Urine output should be monitored hourly and Caesarean section should be considered if labour does not become established fairly quickly. Catheterize the patient and leave the catheter *in situ* to monitor urinary output.
- The longer the fetus stays in the uterus the greater the chance of disseminated intravascular coagulation developing.
- Expect and be prepared for massive postpartum haemorrhage whether the baby is delivered normally or by Caesarean section.
- In cases of severe antepartum haemorrhage requiring surgery, discuss the possibility of hysterectomy with the patient or if appropriate with her designated partner.
- *Remember*: *It is the APH which weakens the patient and then the PPH that kills.*

Suspect and aggressively treat coagulopathy in discussion with haematologist

Give platelets to treat thrombocytopenia. Platelets are transfused when platelets have fallen below $50 \times 10^9/l$ or in massive transfusion (with every 8 units of blood). In the case of dilutional coagulopathy (coagulopathy after 8–10 units of blood where there is no suspicion of DIC, fresh frozen plasma (FFP) provides the clotting factors required and should be given at a rate of 1 unit for every 6 units of rapidly transfused blood or guided by the results of clotting studies.

Give FFP and cryoprecipitate to correct clotting factor deficiencies. Cryoprecipitate is given when fibrinogen levels have fallen to less than 100 units.

SYSTEMATIC REVIEW

Offringa M (1998) Excess mortality after human albumin administration in critically ill patients. *Clinical and pathophysiological evidence suggests albumin is harmful. Br Med J.* **318**: 223–224.

MASSIVE OBSTETRIC HAEMORRHAGE – DIC

Massive obstetric haemorrhage is blood loss in excess of 1000 ml from the genital tract. The loss may be concealed. The 1994–1996 Report on Confidential Enquiries into Maternal Deaths in the United Kingdom found haemorrhage to be the sixth leading cause of death.

Disseminated Intravascular Coagulation (DIC) is a failure of haemostasis which can result in massive haemorrhage. DIC is the result of activation of the coagulation and fibrinolytic systems which leads to deficiencies of coagulation proteins, fibrinogen and platelets. The clinical presentation can be major bleeding with or without thrombotic complications. Hypotension-mediated endothelial injury may trigger DIC. Haemorrhage should be acted upon before hypotension occurs, particularly in the presence of known risk factors.

ACTION PLAN

1 **Suspect**

2 **Call for senior obstetrician, anaesthetist, theatre team, extra midwifery staff and porter to be readily available**

3 **Discuss urgency with haematologist, so that ABO and RhD matched blood can be made available if necessary**

4 **Airway**
- Assess.
- Maintain patency.
- Apply oxygen 15 l/min via tight fitting face mask with reservoir bag.
- Attach pulse oximeter to patient.

Breathing
- Assess.
- Ventilate.
- Protect airway.
- Regularly monitor RR.

Circulation
- CPR if necessary.
- Treat peri-arrest arrhythmias.
- Tilt to left.
- Assess volume loss by overt losses, peripheral perfusion, pulse, blood pressure and catheterize and measure urine output half hourly.
- Remember haemorrhage is invariably underestimated.

5 **Replace volume loss**
- Insert two large bore i.v. cannulae.
- Send bloods for FBC, clotting studies, cross-match 6 units.
- Correct volume loss initially by up to 2 l of normal saline followed by synthetic colloid, then whole blood or packed red cells as soon as they are available.

- If blood loss is life-threatening group O Rh negative red cells should be used if this is the fastest available source of red cells.
- Consider group specific blood but preferably use fully cross-matched blood.
- Warm i.v. fluids.
- Infuse with a pressure bag.
- Consider CVP for monitoring and i.v. access, PCWP and arterial pressure monitoring.
- Move to high dependency area of labour ward.

6 **Correct the cause of DIC**

7 **Suspect and aggressively treat coagulopathy in discussion with haematologist**

8 **If antepartum continuously monitor FH by cardiotocography and consider timing and method of delivery**

9 **Diagnose source of bleeding and treat**

10 **Check FBC, haematocrit clotting and arterial blood gases regularly as appropriate**

11 **Consider transfer to HDU/ICU**

12 **Discuss treatment of embolic phenomena with consultant haematologist**

13 **Keep a record of pulse, BP, RR, SaO$_2$, CVP, PCWP, urine output, fluids given, laboratory results and FH**

14 **Document in the notes with time, date, a signature and printed identification**

CONSULT OTHER TOPICS

SUPPLEMENTARY INFORMATION

Correct the cause of DIC

DIC may be triggered by hypotension in 'uncomplicated' massive obstetric haemorrhage. Specific obstetric causes of DIC include pre-eclampsia, amniotic fluid embolism, placental abruption and intrauterine death. Supportive and definitive treatment as available should be given for individual conditions.

Suspect and aggressively treat coagulopathy in discussion with haematologist

- Give platelets to treat thrombocytopenia. Platelets are transfused when platelets have fallen below $50 \times 10^9/l$ or in massive transfusion.
- Give FFP and cryoprecipitate to correct clotting factor deficiencies. Cryoprecipitate is given when fibrinogen levels have fallen to less than 100 units.

Consider transfer to HDU/ICU

The patient may require intubation and ventilation to be adequately oxygenated. She is at risk of developing adult respiratory distress syndrome (ARDS) and other systems failure.

Discuss treatment of embolic phenomena with consultant haematologist

If fibrinogen depletion is identified, consider the administration of heparin, fibrinogen and fibrinolytic agents, e.g. tranexamic acid.

SYSTEMATIC REVIEW

Offringa M (1998) Excess mortality after human albumin administration in critically ill patients. *Clinical and pathophysiological evidence suggests albumin is harmful.* Br. Med. J. **318**: 223–224.

REFERENCE

McClelland B (ed) (1996) Acquired haemostatic problems. *Handbook of Transfusion Medicine*, 2nd edn. HMSO, London.

MASSIVE OBSTETRIC HAEMORRHAGE – POSTPARTUM

The 1994–1996 Report on Confidential Enquiries into Maternal Deaths in the United Kingdom found haemorrhage to be the sixth leading cause of death. Massive postpartum obstetric haemorrhage is defined as blood loss from the genital tract following delivery, in excess of 1000 ml. The principles of treatment are to replace blood and to control haemorrhage. There may be local guidelines.

ACTION PLAN

1 **Suspect**

2 **Call for senior obstetrician, anaesthetist, theatre team, extra midwifery staff and porter to be readily available**

3 **Discuss urgency with haematologist, so that ABO and RhD matched blood can be made available if necessary**

4 **Airway**
- Assess.
- Maintain patency.
- Apply oxygen 15 l/min via tight fitting face mask with reservoir bag.
- Attach pulse oximeter to patient.

Breathing
- Assess.
- Ventilate.
- Protect airway.
- Regularly monitor RR.

Circulation
- CPR if necessary.
- Treat peri-arrest arrhythmias.
- Assess volume loss by overt losses, peripheral perfusion, pulse, blood pressure and catheterize and measure urine output half hourly.
- Remember haemorrhage is invariably underestimated.

5 **Replace volume loss**
- Insert two large bore i.v. cannulae.
- Send bloods for FBC, clotting studies, cross-match 6 units.
- Correct volume loss initially by up to 2 l of normal saline followed by synthetic colloid, then whole blood or packed red cells as soon as they are available.
- If blood loss is life-threatening group O Rh negative red cells should be used if this is the fastest available source of red cells.
- Consider group-specific blood but preferably use fully cross-matched blood.
- Warm i.v. fluids.
- Infuse with a pressure bag.

- Put on automatic NIBP monitor, consider CVP for monitoring and i.v. access, PCWP and arterial pressure monitoring.
- Move to high dependency area of labour ward.

6 **Diagnose and treat source of bleeding**

7 **Suspect and aggressively treat coagulopathy in discussion with haematologist**

8 **Check FBC, haematocrit, clotting and arterial blood gases regularly as appropriate**

9 **Consider transfer to HDU/ICU**

10 **Keep a record of pulse, BP, RR, SaO$_2$, CVP, PCWP, urine output, fluids given, laboratory results and FH**

11 **Document in the notes with times, date, a signature and printed identification**

CONSULT OTHER TOPICS

Airway obstruction (p. 1)
Caesarean hysterectomy (p. 52)
Cardiopulmonary resuscitation (p. 8)
Hypotension (p. 150)
Inverted uterus (p. 85)
Massive obstetric haemorrhage – DIC (p. 92)
Peri-arrest arrhythmias (p. 16)
Postpartum genital tract trauma (p. 104)
Respiratory emergencies (p. 20)
Retained placenta (p. 116)

SUPPLEMENTARY INFORMATION

Diagnose and treat source of bleeding

Causes

- Atonic or relaxing uterus.
- Retained products.
- Trauma to uterus or birth canal.

Treatment

(a) Rub up a contraction and administer an oxytocic or repeat dose of oxytocic – syntometrine (5 IU of syntocinon and 0.5 mg of ergometrine).
(b) Examine the patient: if analgesia adequate, i.e. good epidural, explore the uterus for retained products and integrity of uterine cavity.
(c) Check for bleeding from the cervix, vaginal walls and perineum. Ensure adequate analgesia.
(d) Reassess. Is bleeding continuing? Is there a clotting disorder?
(e) If bleeding continues, re-examine under anaesthesia; ensure syntocinon drip is running.

(f) Exclude

- inverted uterus,
- retained products,
- damage to genital tract.

(g) Apply bimanual compression.
(h) If bleeding from an empty, apparently undamaged uterus continues give

- Carboprost (Hemabate) 250 µg intramuscular or intramyometrial, maximum dose 2 mg.
- Vasopressin – subendothelial at bleeding site. Serial 1 ml injections 5 IU (1 ml).
- Vasopressin diluted in 19 ml of 0.9% sodium chloride. The injection should not be directly into a blood vessel.
- Prostaglandin pessaries or gel can be placed directly in the uterus.

(i) Intrauterine direct pressure from a balloon hydrostatic/catheter (size 16; available from Rüsch) may be successful (intrauterine packing is not recommended).
(j) Consider arterial embolization under X-ray control.

Surgical treatment

(a) Laparotomy.
(b) Ligation of the internal iliac arteries in continuity at the bifurcation results in 77% reduction in pulse pressure distal to the ligation and controls haemorrhage in approximately 50% of atonic PPHs.
(c) Compression of the uterus using the B-Lynch brace sutures.
(d) Hysterectomy may be life saving and should be considered early to reduce risk of life-threatening coagulopathy; a subtotal hysterectomy may be preferable.
(e) Bleeding continuing after hysterectomy may be controlled by the use of a transvaginal pressure pack. A bag is placed in the pelvis and filled with gauze, the neck of the bag is brought out through the vagina with the ends of the gauze packs to facilitate later removal. A litre bag of fluid can be attached to the end of the bag to apply pressure.

Suspect and aggressively treat coagulopathy in discussion with haematologist

Give platelets to treat thrombocytopenia. Platelets are transfused when platelets have fallen below $50 \times 10^9/l$ or in massive transfusion.

In the case of dilutional coagulopathy (coagulopathy after 8–10 units of blood where there is no suspicion of DIC, fresh frozen plasma (FFP) provides the clotting factors required and should be given at a rate of 1 unit for every 6 units of rapidly transfused blood or guided by the results of clotting studies.

Give FFP and cryoprecipitate to correct clotting factor deficiencies. Cryoprecipitate is given when fibrinogen levels have fallen to less than 100 units.

Severe secondary postpartum haemorrhage is usually caused by retained products which undergo necrosis, become infected and retard involution of the uterus. Adequately resuscitate and initially give antibiotics for 24 hours if possible. Explore the uterus to remove necrotic, possibly infected, retained products of conception. Laparotomy is necessary only rarely to deal with continued bleeding from an infected or ruptured uterine incision or infected placental bed. Massive postpartum haemorrhage may cause pituitary infarction – Sheehan's syndrome, Simmonds disease.

SYSTEMATIC REVIEWS

Gulmezoglu AM (1999) Prostaglandins for prevention of postpartum haemorrhage (Cochrane Review). *The Cochrane Library*, Issue 2. Update Software, Oxford.

Reviewers' conclusions: *Although injectable prostaglandins appear to be effective in preventing postpartum haemorrhage, concerns about safety and costs limit their suitability for routine prophylactic management of the third stage of labour. However, injectable prostaglandins should continue to be used for the treatment of postpartum haemorrhage when other measures fail. Misoprostol is cheap, stable and seems to be safe. Trials addressing the effectiveness of misoprostol are continuing.*

Offringa M (1999) Excess mortality after human albumin administration in critically ill patients. *Clinical and pathophysiological evidence suggests albumin is harmful.* Br. Med. J. **318**: 223–224.

PERIPARTUM CARDIOMYOPATHY

Peripartum cardiomyopathy is a rare cause of peripartum heart failure and is of unknown aetiology. It is a life-threatening condition and has a maternal mortality of 25–50%. Other causes of heart failure must be excluded.

ACTION PLAN

1 **Suspect**

2 **Diagnosis**
- Development of cardiac failure in the last month of pregnancy or within 5 months of delivery.
- Absence of a determinable cause for cardiac failure.
- Absence of demonstrable heart disease before the last month of pregnancy.
- Echocardiographically demonstrable impairment in left ventricular systolic function.

3 **Airway**
- Assess.
- Maintain patency.
- Apply oxygen 15 l/min via tight fitting face mask with reservoir bag.
- Attach pulse oximeter to patient.
- Call anaesthetist if SaO_2 < 94% on oxygen.

Breathing
- Consider elective tracheal intubation, ventilation and PEEP if necessary.

Circulation
- Assess pulse and BP.
- CPR if necessary.
- Tilt to left.
- Put on ECG and automatic BP monitor.
- Treat peri-arrest arrhythmias.
- Secure i.v. access, send bloods for FBC, U&Es, group and save.

4 **Call cardiologists**

5 **Consider invasive monitoring if haemodynamically unstable or respiratory compromise**

6 **Request CXR and ECG**

7 **Treat with digoxin, diuretics, ACE inhibitors and vasodilators**

8 **Restrict sodium intake**

9 **Consider anticoagulation**

10 **Monitor FH by continuous cardiotocography and consider timing and method of delivery if antepartum**

11 **Keep a record of pulse, BP, RR, SaO$_2$, CVP, FH if appropriate and treatments given**

12 **Transfer to ICU**

13 **Consider immunosuppression**

14 **Consider cardiac transplant**

15 **Document findings, treatments and management plan in notes, with time, date, a signature and printed identification**

16 **Provide counselling as to the advisability of future pregnancies**

CONSULT OTHER TOPICS

Acute abdominal pain (p. 44)
Acute chest pain (p. 128)
Airway obstruction (p. 1)
Amniotic fluid embolism (p. 47)
Cardiopulmonary resuscitation (p. 8)
Eclampsia, pre-eclampsia, HELLP, fatty liver and hepatic rupture (p. 66)
Hypertension (p. 147)
Hypotension (p. 150)
Peri-arrest arrhythmias (p. 16)
Respiratory emergencies (p. 20)
Substance abuse (p. 173)
Thromboembolism (p. 177)
Twins and multiple pregnancies (p. 122)

SUPPLEMENTARY INFORMATION

Suspect

Symptoms and signs are dyspnoea, cough, orthopnoea, paroxysmal nocturnal dyspnoea, fatigue, palpitations, haemoptysis, chest pain, abdominal pain, normal or increased blood pressure, increased JVP, cardiomegaly, third heart sound, loud second heart sound, mitral or tricuspid regurgitation, peripheral oedema, ascites, arrhythmias, embolic phenomena and hepatomegaly.

Risk factors

- Advanced maternal age.
- Multiparity.
- Twin pregnancy.
- African descent.
- Long-term tocolytic therapy.
- Cocaine abuse possibly.

Diagnosis

Suspect if worsening symptoms of heart failure in late pregnancy or early puerperium. Peripartum cardiomyopathy is rarely seen before 36 weeks' gestation. Heart failure from other causes usually presents in the second trimester of pregnancy.

Treat with digoxin, diuretics, ACE inhibitors and vasodilators

- Specific treatment should be given in consultation with consultant cardiologist.
- Digoxin is beneficial for its effects on ventricular contractility and rate control.
- Diuretics are fundamental in the treatment of heart failure and provide good symptomatic relief.
- Vasodilators reduce afterload and allow an improvement in cardiac output.
- ACE inhibitors are contraindicated in pregnancy but are useful in those with peripartum cardiomyopathy which occurs in the early postpartum months. Breastfeeding should be discouraged in patients who require ACE inhibitor therapy, i.e. those with persistent left ventricular dysfunction.
- When vasodilator therapy is required prepartum, hydrallazine is the drug of choice.

Consider anticoagulation

Thromboembolic phenomena may occur in up to 53% of cases. Before delivery heparin is the drug of choice. Bed rest is not recommended.

Transfer to ICU

Invasive monitoring and intense supportive therapy are required. Prognosis is related to the recovery of left ventricular function.

Consider immunosuppression

Immunosupression has been recommended for patients with peripartum cardio-myopathy and myocarditis diagnosed by biopsy.

Consider cardiac transplant

Cardiac transplantation has been performed successfully. Cardiopulmonary bypass may be necessary whilst awaiting a donor heart. These patients have a higher rejection/infection rate than patients with idiopathic cardiomyopathy.

Provide counselling as to the advisability of future pregnancies

Patients with persistent left ventricular dysfunction (as demonstrated by echo-cardiography) are at very high risk of complications and death should they become pregnant again. Caution is recommended to patient initially and further investigation and discussion with cardiologist should be undertaken.

REFERENCE

Lampert MB and Lang RM (1995) Peripartum cardiomyopathy. *Am. Heart J.* **130**: 860–870.

Peripartum Cardiomyopathy

PLACENTA ACCRETA/PERCRETA

E. O'Donnell

This is defined as morbid adherence of the placenta. Over the past 40 years, the incidence of placenta accreta has increased 10-fold. This is related to the increase in Caesarean section rates. The initial presentation is as a retained placenta. It becomes apparent however, during manual removal that complete placental separation cannot be achieved.

1 **Airway**
- Assess.
- Maintain patency.
- Apply oxygen 15 l/min via tight fitting face mask with reservoir bag.
- Attach pulse oximeter to patient.
- Call anaesthetist.

Breathing
- Assess.
- Ventilate.
- Protect airway.

Circulation
- Assess pulse and BP.
- CPR.
- Tilt to left.
- Put on ECG and BP monitor.
- Treat peri-arrest arrhythmias.
- Secure i.v. access with large bore cannula.
- Send bloods for FBC, U&Es and cross-match.
- Replace intravascular volume, with blood if necessary.

2 **If placenta accreta is suspected obtain consent which should include possible hysterectomy**

3 **Call senior obstetrician**

4 **If there is sustained adequate haemostasis manage conservatively and prescribe prophylactic antibiotics**

5 **If there is haemorrhage an exploratory laparotomy will be required**

6 **If the woman has completed her family, hysterectomy is the treatment of choice**

7 **Conservative measures are only appropriate if the women is haemodynamically stable and future childbearing is an overwhelming concern**

8 **Document findings, treatment and management plan in the notes with time, date, a signature and printed identification**

CONSULT OTHER TOPICS

Acute abdominal pain (p. 44)
Airway obstruction (p. 1)
Caesarean section – complications (p. 55)
Cardiopulmonary resuscitation (p. 8)
Hypotension (p. 150)
Massive obstetric haemorrhage – postpartum (p. 95)
Peri-arrest arrhythmias (p. 16)
Respiratory emergencies (p. 20)
Retained placenta (p. 116)

SUPPLEMENTARY INFORMATION

If there is sustained adequate haemostasis manage conservatively and prescribe prophylactic antibiotics

Conservative management of placenta accreta is associated with high rates of secondary infection and therefore prophylactic antibiotics are mandatory until uterine involution has occurred. Conservative treatment may be successful in 50% of women.

Conservative measures are only appropriate if the women is haemodynamically stable and future childbearing is an overwhelming concern

Conservative treatment options include placental bed diathermy, 'figure of eight' sutures, oxytocic drugs including haemabate, vessel ligation, or placental bed tamponade, e.g. using a Sengstaken–Blakemore tube filled with 200 ml of saline, and angiographic embolization.

REFERENCES

Clarke SL, Koonings P and Phelan JP (1984) Placenta accreta and previous cesarean section. *Obstet. Gynecol.* **66**: 89.
Weckstein LN, Masserman JS and Garite TJ (1987) Placenta accreta: a problem of increasing clinical significance. *Obstet. Gynecol.* **69**: 480.

Placenta Accreta/Percreta

POSTPARTUM GENITAL TRACT TRAUMA

Genital tract trauma refers to damage to the cervix, vagina, paravaginal or paragenital tissues, perineum, urethra, bladder, anus or rectum. Action plans for all these are given below.

The perineum should be inspected for obvious bleeding points which should be secured either by haemostats or by suturing. It is unwise however to suture the perineum without excluding haemorrhage or damage higher up. Appropriate analgesia or anaesthesia should be provided for an adequate examination of the genital tract.

CERVIX

ACTION PLAN

1 **Suspect**

2 **After securing obvious bleeders in the perineum, inspect the vagina and cervix**
- A good light and an assistant are essential.

3 **Place a weighted speculum in the vagina and expose the cervix**
- The cervix often looks damaged but rarely bleeds.

4 **To examine the cervix properly side wall retractors or 2 Sim's speculi are needed**
- The cervix should be grasped by sponge forceps and these should be moved around the cervix one at a time so that the whole of the cervix can be examined circumferentially.

5 **If a bleeding point is identified then the apex of the tear must be identified before suturing**

6 **Deeper lacerations may involve the vaginal vault and may extend towards the bladder or out towards the uterine artery at the base of the broad ligament and can lead to severe haemorrhage which requires laparotomy**

VAGINA

ACTION PLAN

1 **Suspect**

2 **Be aware a common cause of continued postpartum haemorrhage is from the apex of a vaginal tear which has not been reached at the time of repair of episiotomy or tear**

3 **Adequate exposure is necessary and it is often necessary to take down the existing repair to carry out an adequate examination**
- A suture should be placed as high up the laceration as possible then used as a retractor to pull the apex into view so that it can be secured.

PARAVAGINAL OR PARAGENITAL HAEMATOMA

1 **Suspect**
   - If the patient collapses at some time after the third stage of labour with signs of shock in the absence of external haemorrhage.

2 **Subsequent management depends on whether the bleeding (which is external to the walls of the genital tract) is coming from above or below the levator ani muscle**

3 **A vulval haematoma lies *below* the levator ani, is usually obvious and usually requires evacuation in addition to resuscitation**
   - Incise through the vagina to minimize scarring.
   - Achieve haemostasis by evacuating the clot, direct pressure and the use of figure of eight sutures.
   - If oozing continues a pack can be placed in the cavity or the wound can be closed and drained.

4 **A subperitoneal/broad ligament haematoma lies *above* the levator ani**
   - One third occur after spontaneous vaginal delivery, one third after forceps delivery and one third after caesarean section.
   - Inform a senior obstetrician.
   - Adopt a conservative approach if haemodynamically stable.
   - If haemodynamically unstable, perform a laparotomy.
   - Before proceeding to laparotomy, obtain consent for hysterectomy.

URETHRA

1 **Suspect**

2 **If urethral damage is suspected consult a senior obstetrician**

3 **Inspect urethra and anterior vaginal wall and pass a catheter**
   - If there is only blood or a small amount of blood-stained urine the catheter should be left *in situ* and urine output monitored carefully.

4 **Repair any obvious lacerations to the urethra over the catheter and leave the catheter *in situ* for at least 7 days**

5 **Make a follow-up appointment**

BLADDER

1 Suspect

2 Examine the upper anterior wall of the bladder

3 If there is a laceration into the bladder through the upper wall of the anterior vagina this should be assessed by a senior obstetrician

4 The ureters need to be identified and catheterized before repair is undertaken

5 The repair should be in two layers and the two layers closed in different directions to avoid the two stitch lines lying directly over each other

6 The bladder should be drained for 10–14 days

7 At Caesarean section damage to the bladder is easily missed until after the baby has been delivered

8 If the bladder is damaged a senior obstetrician should be consulted

9 The bladder should be repaired in two layers using absorbable sutures

10 Give antibiotic cover

11 Ensure a good urinary output

URETER

1 Suspect

2 A senior obstetrician should attend and the opinion of a urologist will usually be requested if ureteric damage is suspected

3 The damage is likely to be near the uterus and reimplantation is likely to be the operation of choice if the ureter is divided or badly damaged

4 The patient needs to be followed up and an intravenous urogram carried out to check for stenosis or reflux

EPISIOTOMY OR PERINEAL TEAR

ACTION PLAN

1 Ensure that there is adequate analgesia

2 Examine for other lacerations involving the urethra or upper vagina

3 Ensure that anal sphincter is intact

4 Ensure that the apex of the episiotomy is identified and that the first bite of the suture secures it

5 Suture the vagina with a continuous polyglycolic stitch

6 Use deep tension free polyglycolic sutures either interrupted or continuous to the muscle layer

7 Suture perineal skin subcuticularly to minimize discomfort

8 Perform rectal examination to ensure that sutures have not passed into the rectal lumen and the lumen is not occluded

9 The swabs should be counted

THIRD OR FOURTH DEGREE TEARS

ACTION PLAN

1 Suspect if the episiotomy or tear extends

2 To carry out an adequate repair either a general anaesthetic or a regional block is required

3 The repair must be carried out by an experienced obstetrician

4 The episiotomy or tear is repaired in the normal way but the tear in the anal sphincter should be by the overlapping method and a monofilament suture rather than a braided suture should be used

- End to end repair using a figure of eight suture has an unsatisfactory outcome.

5 Ensure careful haemostasis and give antibiotic cover intraoperatively using augmentin or cephradine and metronidazole

- Haematoma formation and infection frequently lead to breakdown and failure of the repair.

6 Careful follow-up should be arranged to monitor outcome

- Further investigations such as anorectal ultrasound may need to be arranged.

Postpartum Genital Tract Trauma

CONSULT OTHER TOPICS

SUPPLEMENTARY INFORMATION

Suspect

Suspect where there is obvious perineal disruption, continued bleeding with a contracted uterus or apparent hypovolaemic shock in the absence of external haemorrhage. It may be difficult to identify the source of haemorrhage as a certain amount of bleeding can be expected to come from the cavity of the uterus.

The urethra and bladder are commonly contused during delivery, either spontaneous or assisted. More serious damage can occur during rotational forceps deliveries (especially if catheterization of the bladder has inadvertently been omitted), Caesarean section and neglected labours.

Suspect if there has been prolonged labour and the urine is blood-stained, if there has been a difficult forceps delivery (especially rotational) or if there has been a suspicion of bladder or ureteric damage at Caesarean section.

Third or fourth degree tears

The UK definition is any disruption of the anal sphincter irrespective of anal epithelial involvement; 35% of primipara sustain occult anal sphincter injuries.

Routine episiotomy does not reduce the rate of anal sphincter damage either in those who have not delivered vaginally before or those who have sustained previous damage.

If a patient has had a third degree tear, Caesarean section is likely to be a better option if anorectal physiology tests and anorectal ultrasound suggests significant sphincter defects.

SYSTEMATIC REVIEWS

Kettle C and Johanson RB (1999) Absorbable synthetic versus catgut suture for perineal repair (Cochrane Review). *The Cochrane Library*, Issue 2. Update Software, Oxford.

Reviewers' conclusions: *Absorbable synthetic suture material (in the form of polyglycolic acid sutures) for perineal repair following childbirth appears to decrease women's experience of short-term pain. The length of time taken for the synthetic material to be absorbed is of concern. A trial addressing the use of polyglactin has recently been completed and will be included in the next version of this review.*

Kettle C and Johanson RB (1999) Continuous versus interrupted sutures for perineal repair (Cochrane Review). *The Cochrane Library*, Issue 2. Update Software, Oxford.

Postpartum Genital Tract Trauma

Reviewers' conclusions: *The continuous subcuticular technique of perineal repair may be associated with less pain in the immediate postpartum period than the interrupted suture technique. The long-term effects are less clear.*

REFERENCES

Londono-Schimmer EE, Garcia-Duperly R, Nicholls RJ, Ritchie JK, Hawley PR and Thompson JPS (1994) Overlapping anal sphincter repair for faecal incontinence due to sphincter trauma: five year follow-up functional results. *Int. J. Colorect. Dis.* **9**: 110–113.

Neilsen MB, Hauge C, Raamussen OO, Petersen JF and Christiansen J (1992) Anal endoscopic findings in the follow-up of primary sutured sphincteric ruptures. *Br. J. Surg.* **79**: 104–106.

Sultan AH, Kamm MA, Bartram CI and Hudson CN (1994) Perineal damage at delivery. *Contemp. Rev. Obstet. Gynaecol.* **6**: 18–24.

PREMATURE LABOUR

Premature labour is defined as the onset of regular uterine contractions, with or without rupture of membranes, resulting in changes in the state of the cervix, occurring before 37 completed weeks of gestation. The diagnosis of premature labour is essentially retrospective! The incidence is between 5 and 10%.

1 **Assess or reassess gestation**

2 **Search for a cause**

3 **Administer parenteral steroids if the patient is between 24 and 36 weeks of gestation**

4 **Consider the use of tocolytics**

5 **Check that a cot is available in a particular unit if the pre-term fetus delivers, consider transfer if not, but not if the labour appears to be progressing quickly**

6 **Check whether the membranes are intact**

7 **Check the presentation of the fetus and formulate a delivery plan**

8 **If very preterm ask the paediatrician to see the mother to discuss the likely prognosis which may well affect decision with regard to mode of delivery**

9 **Document assessment, decisions and management plan clearly in notes with date, time, a signature and printed identification**

CONSULT OTHER TOPICS

Abnormal presentations and positions – breech (p. 34)
Intrauterine death (p. 81)
Massive obstetric haemorrhage – antepartum (p. 88)
Neonatal resuscitation (p. 14)
Puerperal sepsis, septicaemia and septic shock (p. 113)
Risk management (p. 185)
Twins and multiple pregnancies (p. 122)

SUPPLEMENTARY INFORMATION

Assess or reassess gestation

Check that the pregnancy is 34 or more weeks' gestation. If so the labour should be allowed to progress. Gestation should be confirmed by reassessment of menstrual dates and early ultrasound scans.

Risk factors

- First pregnancy.
- Extremes of childbearing years.
- Deprived socioeconomic environment.
- Smoking.
- Unsupported mother.
- Stress.
- Previous premature delivery or midtrimester pregnancy loss.
- Antepartum haemorrhage in this pregnancy.
- Multiple pregnancy and polyhydramnios.
- Uterine malformations.
- Fetal abnormalities.
- Severe maternal illnesses.
- Genital tract infections especially bacterial vaginosis.

Search for a cause

If placental abruption or chorioamnionitis is suspected then tocolytic therapy is contraindicated.

Administer parenteral steroids if the patient is between 24 and 36 weeks of gestation

These are the Royal College of Obstetricians and Gynaecologists' guidelines.

Dexamethasone 12 mg is given immediately intramuscularly, and 12 hours later a further 12 mg dose is administered. There is a risk of using steroids in patients with intrauterine infection or diabetic patients who have had difficulty in controlling their diabetes. Recent animal work has shown that the repeated use of steroids in pregnancy may affect the development of the fetal brain and follow-up studies have shown no significant long-term benefits over the one-off steroid regime.

Consider the use of tocolytics

Ritodrine and salbutamol are the commonest agents to be used and may delay delivery by up to 1 week. This will allow fetal lung maturity to progress. Tocolytics are not widely used at present, with the exception of patients who may need to be transferred for delivery to another hospital, as they are not of proven benefit in preterm labour.

Nifedipine, indomethacin, magnesium sulphate and nitrates are also being used.

Check the presentation of the fetus and formulate a delivery plan

Malpresentations such as breech are much more likely in premature infants. Many obstetricians would favour Caesarean section for the delivery of the premature breech or multiple pregnancy.

SYSTEMATIC REVIEWS

Crowley P (1999) Prophylactic corticosteroids for preterm delivery (Cochrane Review). *The Cochrane Library*, Issue 2. Update Software, Oxford.

Reviewers' conclusions: *Corticosteroids given prior to preterm birth (as a result of either preterm labour or elective preterm delivery) are effective in preventing respiratory distress syndrome and neonatal mortality. However there is not enough evidence to evaluate the use of repeated doses of corticosteroid in women who remain undelivered, but who are at continued risk of preterm birth.*

Crowther CA and Moore V (1999) Magnesium for preventing preterm birth after threatened preterm labour (Cochrane Review). *The Cochrane Library*, Issue 2. Update Software, Oxford.

Reviewers' conclusions: *There is not enough evidence to show that magnesium maintenance therapy is effective in preventing preterm birth after an episode of threatened preterm labour.*

Grant A (1999) Elective versus selective Caesarean section for delivery of the small baby (Cochrane Review). *The Cochrane Library*, Issue 2. Update Software, Oxford.

Reviewers' conclusions: *There is not enough evidence to evaluate the use of a policy for elective Caesarean delivery for small babies. Randomized trials in this area are likely to continue to experience recruitment problems. However it still may be possible to investigate elective Caesarean delivery in preterm babies presenting cephalically.*

PUERPERAL SEPSIS, SEPTICAEMIA AND SEPTIC SHOCK

E. O'Donnell and K. Grady

Septic shock causes inadequate tissue perfusion and ultimately multiorgan failure. It results from overwhelming sepsis.

In 1984 the American College of Obstetricians and Gynaecologists suggested that a preliminary diagnosis of septic shock should be made when there is hypotension preceded by pyrexia. Other features of the condition may include hypoxia, cardiovascular collapse, tachycardia, tachypnoea, oliguria and confusion.

Sepsis was one of the five causes which accounted for 85% of maternal deaths in the Report on Confidential Enquiries into Maternal Deaths in the United Kingdom 1994–1996. Aggressive prompt management is required.

ACTION PLAN

1 **Airway**
- Assess.
- Maintain patency.
- Apply oxygen 15 l/min via tight fitting face mask with reservoir bag.
- Attach pulse oximeter to patient.
- Call anaesthetist.
- Consider tracheal intubation.

   Breathing
- Assess.
- Ventilate.
- Protect airway.

   Circulation
- Assess pulse, BP and peripheral perfusion.
- CPR if necessary.
- Put on ECG and automatic BP monitor.
- Treat peri-arrest arhythmias.
- Secure i.v. access with large bore cannula, send bloods for FBC, U&Es, blood cultures and group and save.
- Consider need for CVP line.
- Start i.v. volume expansion with crystalloid or colloid.

2 **Continuously monitor FH by cardiotocography and consider timing and method of delivery**

3 **Call for senior obstetrician**

4 **Consider diagnosis of septic shock and if appropriate invasively monitor**

5 **Consider transfer to HDU/ICU if appropriate**

6 **Consider the use of ionotropes**

7 **Take arterial blood gases** and in discussion with anaesthetist consider bicarbonate for treatment of acidosis

8 **Attempt to establish a focus of infection and treat any obvious source**

9 **Consult microbiologist early and give antibiotics as advised**

10 **Monitoring for and treat complications**

11 **Keep a record to include pulse, BP, RR, SaO$_2$, temperature, CVP, FH and treatments given**

12 **Document findings, diagnosis and treatment in notes, with time, date, a signature and a printed identification**

CONSULT OTHER TOPICS

Airway obstruction (p. 1)
Anaphylaxis (p. 133)
Cardiopulmonary resuscitation (p. 8)
Hypotension (p. 150)
Peri-arrest arrhythmias (p. 16)
Respiratory emergencies (p. 20)

SUPPLEMENTARY INFORMATION

Consider diagnosis of septic shock and if appropriate invasively monitor

If hypotension does not respond to initial fluid bolus of 500 ml the cause may be septic shock. If the clinical picture is suggestive of this, i.e. pyrexia, tachycardia, hyperdynamic peripheral circulation, wide pulse pressure, and hypotension, invasive monitoring of arterial, central venous and pulmonary artery pressures may be appropriate to optimize volume replacement and allow the use of ionotropes.

Consider transfer to HDU/ICU if appropriate

This may be for ventilation or monitoring purposes. Pulmonary artery pressure monitoring is normally only carried out on HDU/ICU. Transfer out of the delivery suite may not be possible, however, for obstetric management.

Consider the use of ionotropes

Septic shock may cause a fall in systemic vascular resistance and myocardial depression resulting in a fall in cardiac output as seen by pulmonary artery flotation catheter measurements. Ionotropes can be used to correct these haemodynamics.

Take arterial blood gases

Inadequate tissue perfusion leads to tissue hypoxia and lactic acid production. Sodium bicarbonate 8.4% should be considered in increments of 50 ml where the base excess is found to be −3 or more.

Attempt to establish a focus of infection and treat any obvious source

The cause of most infections during pregnancy, delivery or the postnatal period can be identified. It is imperative that any infective or necrotic foci, e.g. retained products of conception, be identified and eradicated.

Tests include blood cultures, midstream urine microscopy and culture, throat, vaginal and endocervical swabs, full blood count and differential white cell count, blood film, specific antibody titres, and chest X-rays.

Consult microbiologist early and give antibiotics as advised

Antibiotic therapy should be on the advice of your local microbiologist. This will include preliminary broad spectrum coverage until culture results are available.

Monitor for and treat complications

Consider acute renal failure, respiratory failure, disseminated intravascular coagulation.

REFERENCES

American College of Obstetricians and Gynaecologists (1984) *Septic Shock technical bulletin*, **75**. ACOG, Washington, DC.
Lee W (1989) Management of septic shock complicating pregnancy. *Obstet. Gynecol. Clin. North Am.* **16(2)**: 431–47.

RETAINED PLACENTA

E. O'Donnell and K. Grady

A placenta may be defined as retained if it cannot be expelled within 30 minutes of delivery. The incidence of retained placenta varies with gestational age. At term, the incidence of retained placenta is 2%. Delivery before 26 weeks gestation carries a 20-fold increase risk of retained placenta. With the use of oxytocic drugs and controlled cord traction the third stage is completed in 14 minutes in 90% of term labours. There is no significant increase in haemorrhage until the third stage exceeds 30 minutes. Despite this, if there is non-traumatic bleeding prompt measures to remove the placenta are required regardless of the time interval from delivery.

ACTION PLAN

1 **Airway**
- Assess.
- Maintain patency.
- Apply oxygen 15 l/min via tight fitting face mask with reservoir bag.
- Attach pulse oximeter to patient.
- Call anaesthetist.

   Breathing
- Assess.
- Ventilate.
- Protect airway.

   Circulation
- Assess pulse and BP.
- CPR.
- Put on ECG and automatic BP monitor.
- Treat peri-arrest arrhythmias.
- Secure i.v. access with large bore cannulae and send bloods for FBC, U&Es and cross-match.
- Treat hypotension with intravascular volume replacement.

2 **Catheterize the patient**

3 **Avoid excessive controlled cord traction**

4 **Ensure there are adequate uterine contractions**

5 **Take consent for possible hysterectomy**

6 **Inform the anaesthetist if not already present**

7 **Arrange prompt transfer to theatre**

8 **Check that the placenta is not in the cervical canal or vagina prior to administering an anaesthetic**

9 **Give prophylactic antibiotics**

10 **Carry out manual removal** – call for senior help if accreta and/ or heavy bleeding

11 **Check that the placenta is complete**

12 **Check for vaginal, cervical and uterine trauma**

13 **Document findings and procedure in the notes with time, date, a signature and printed identification**

CONSULT OTHER TOPICS

Airway obstruction (p. 1)
Cardiopulmonary resuscitation (p. 8)
Hypotension (p. 150)
Inverted uterus (p. 85)
Massive obstetric haemorrhage – postpartum (p. 95)
Peri-arrest arrhythmias (p. 16)
Placenta accreta/percreta (p. 102)
Respiratory emergencies (p. 20)

SUPPLEMENTARY INFORMATION

Avoid excessive controlled cord traction

If the placenta does not separate readily do not use excessive cord traction as this may result in uterine inversion. Signs of placental separation include lengthening of the cord, fresh bleeding, rise in height of the fundus and increased uterine mobility.

Ensure there are adequate uterine contractions

If the uterus is not contracted, rub up a contraction, put the baby to the breast or give an oxytocic agent. If the placenta fails to deliver within 30 min or if there is excessive bleeding prompt action is required.

If the uterus is well contracted then the placenta is probably separated but trapped in the cervix. If this is the case wait for the cervix to relax and then release the placenta.

Arrange prompt transfer to theatre

Manual removal requires analgesia in the form of general, spinal or epidural anaesthesia.

Give prophylactic antibiotics

Antibiotics should be routinely administered as there is a significant association between manual removal and endometritis.

Carry out manual removal

Under asepsis with the mother in lithotomy position, the uterus is stabilized abdominally with one hand. The other hand (wearing a gauntlet glove) is inserted into the uterus and the placental site is located by following the cord. The placenta is separated from the uterus using the ulnar border of your hand. When the placenta is separated in its entirety it can be removed by controlled cord traction.

Retained Placenta

117

SYSTEMATIC REVIEW

Carroli G and Bergel E (1999) Umbilical vein injection for management of retained placenta (Cochrane Review). *The Cochrane Library*, Issue 2. Update Software, Oxford.

Reviewers' conclusions: *Umbilical vein injection of saline solution plus oxytocin appears to be effective in the management of retained placenta. Saline solution alone does not appear to be more effective than expectant management. Further research into umbilical vein injection of oxytocin or prostaglandins is warranted.*

REFERENCES

Combs CA and Laros RK Jr (1991) Prolonged third stage of labour: morbidity and risk factors. *Obstet. Gynecol.* **77**: 863.

Dombrowski MP, Bottoms SF and Saleh AAA (1995) Third stage of labour: analysis of duration and clinical practice. *Am. J. Obstet. Gynecol.* **172(4)**: 1279–1284.

SHOULDER DYSTOCIA

Shoulder dystocia is defined as the arrest of spontaneous delivery due to the impaction of the anterior shoulder against the symphysis pubis. The risks to the mother are

- postpartum haemorrhage,
- perineal trauma,
- uterine rupture.

The risks to the fetus are

- hypoxia,
- fractures (clavicle, humerus),
- brachial plexus damage.

ACTION PLAN

1 **Suspect**

2 **Call for help including senior obstetrician, anaesthetist and paediatrician**

3 **Draw buttocks to the edge of bed**

4 **Episiotomy**

5 **Knees to chest** (hyperflexing – McRobert's manoeuvre)

6 **Suprapubic pressure and moderate traction**

7 **Deliver posterior arm and shoulder**

8 **Wood's screw manoeuvre**

9 **On all fours**

10 **If all the above fail, try symphysiotomy, cleidotomy or Zavanelli manoeuvre**

11 **Carefully examine the genital tract for damage after delivery**

12 **Document delivery fully in notes with date, time, a signature and printed identification**

13 **Consider risk management issues**

CONSULT OTHER TOPICS

Shoulder Dystocia

SUPPLEMENTARY INFORMATION

Suspect

During pregnancy

- Macrosomia.
- Previous dystocia or big baby.
- Diabetes.
- Prolonged gestation.
- High maternal birth weight.

Write in the notes – BIG BABY: BEWARE SHOULDER DYSTOCIA.

During labour

- Slow progress in the first stage of labour.
- Secondary arrest after 8 cm.
- Midcavity arrest.
- Need for midcavity assisted delivery.

Beware the multiparous patient making slow progress, especially in the second stage.

During delivery

- Head delivering at the end of a contraction.
- Difficulty with delivery of face and chin.
- Retraction of head between contractions – 'turtle necking'.
- A request for assistance by the midwife.

However, it is unpredictable – 50% of dystocia occurs in normal size babies, 98% of macrosomic babies do not have dystocia.

Episiotomy

This is recommended to allow more room for manoeuvres like delivering the posterior shoulder. It allows the operator to use the hollow of the sacrum for such manoeuvres. It reduces the incidence of vaginal lacerations.

Episiotomy should be mediolateral if not already made or consider extending existing one.

Knees to chest (hyperflexing – McRobert's manoeuvre)

Both thighs are sharply flexed against the abdomen. This position serves to straighten the sacrum relative to the lumbar vertebrae and causes cephalic rotation of the pelvis to occur, which helps free the impacted shoulder. This manoeuvre reduces the amount of traction needed and, subsequently, brachial plexus injuries and clavicle fractures. Patients should be put in McRobert's position before applying traction to the fetal neck.

Hips are hyperflexed to open up pelvis. This can also be done by adopting the left lateral with knees to chest position.

Suprapubic pressure and moderate traction

Suprapubic pressure is applied in a posterolateral direction towards the baby's face to encourage the shoulder to rotate under the pubic bone. At the same time head and neck should be pushed downwards. Avoid strong rotational and posterior pressure and sudden changes in force. Indiscriminate pressure on the fundus is associated with risk of damage to fetus and uterus.

Deliver posterior arm and shoulder

The hand of the operator should be passed up to the fetal axilla and the shoulder hooked down – there is always more room in the hollow of the sacrum. Traction on the posterior axilla usually enables the operator to bring down the posterior arm within reach. The posterior arm can then be delivered or if the cubital fossa is within reach, backward pressure on it will result in disengagement of the arm which can then be gently brought down. This is achieved by getting hold of the hand and sweeping it across the chest.

Wood's screw manoeuvre

If delivering the posterior shoulder is not successful, this manoeuvre is applied which involves rotation of the posterior shoulder 180 degrees in a corkscrew fashion in a clockwise or anticlockwise direction so that the impacted anterior shoulder can be released. It is important not to twist the fetal head or neck.

On all fours

This increases the anterposterior diameter of the inlet and facilitates other manoeuvres.

If the above fail, try symphysiotomy, cleidotomy or Zavanelli manoeuvre

Symphysiotomy

This requires inserting a urethral catheter to move the urethra to one side. Two assistants support the legs after taking them out of the stirrups. An incomplete midline cut in the symphyseal joint is made. This, in addition to an episiotomy, will increase the space available and facilitate the delivery of the shoulders.

Cleidotomy

Because of the risk to the fetal subclavian artery the clavicle would only be cut if the baby is dead. There is also risk of maternal trauma.

Zavanelli manoeuvre

This is the reversal of the delivery process by rotating, flexing and reinserting the head into the vagina, followed by Caesarean section. Tocolysis may be needed.

Consider risk management issues

(a) Identify high risk pregnancies antenatally and record this boldly and clearly in the notes.
(b) Discuss fully with mother and document discussion. Inform senior obstetrician and document this in notes.
(c) Assess progress of labour – recognize increased risk if delay.
(d) Have protocol immediately to hand on the labour ward.
(e) Organize practice sessions for midwives and doctors.
(f) After the event, document actions carried out in sequence and timings.
(g) Discuss events with paediatricians and parents.
(h) Inform consultant, senior midwife and risk manager.
(i) Visit mother and baby in the postpartum period.

Shoulder Dystocia

TWINS AND MULTIPLE PREGNANCIES

All obstetric complications are increased, especially the risks to the second or subsequent baby.

There is no convincing evidence that the method of delivery has any effect on neonatal mortality or subsequent neonatal development of low birthweight twins.

ACTION PLAN

1 **Assess and monitor antenatally**

2 **The labour should be managed by an experienced obstetrician with anaesthetic cover immediately available**

3 **Secure intravenous access**

4 **Advise epidural analgesia**

5 **Syntocinon should be available for the second stage**

6 **If first baby is cephalic, e.g. cephalic/cephalic, deliver as if a singleton**

7 **Check fetal heart of the second twin and continually monitor if possible**

8 **Confirm the lie of the second twin, with ultrasound if necessary**

9 **Record the time of delivery of the first twin**

10 **If the lie of the second twin is transverse attempt external cephalic version without delay**

11 **If external cephalic version is successful carry out an artificial rupture of the membranes (ARM) and allow normal vaginal delivery if no fetal distress**

12 **If external cephalic version is unsuccessful either carry out internal podalic version and breech extraction or perform a Caesarean section**

13 **If an internal podalic version and breech extraction is contemplated consult a senior obstetrician**

14 **Carry out assisted delivery of the second twin if there is delay or fetal distress. The ventouse is preferred if the fetus presents cephalically**

15 **If second twin not delivered in 30 minutes inform senior obstetrician and consider caesarean section**

16 **Locked twins are very uncommon and are delivered by Caesarean section, as are the even rarer conjoined twins**

17 Be aware of increased risk of postpartum haemorrhage

18 Make a clear record in notes of method of delivery

CONSULT OTHER TOPICS

Abnormal presentations and positions (p. 34)
Instrumental delivery – forceps (p. 75)
Instrumental delivery – ventouse (p. 78)
Massive obstetric haemorrhage – postpartum (p. 95)

SUPPLEMENTARY INFORMATION

Assess and monitor antenatally

- Presentation of the twins should be confirmed with ultrasound regularly during the pregnancy and on admission in labour.
- The analgesia available for labour should be discussed during pregnancy, ideally with an obstetric anaesthetist. Epidural analgesia is the preferred option.
- If the first baby is breech consider a Caesarean section.
- The option of a planned Caesarean section should be discussed, in particular the possibility of Caesarean section for the second twin after the vaginal birth of the first.
- A decision with regard to the duration of the pregnancy should be made in consultation with the mother taking into account the growth and wellbeing of the babies.
- If twins are thought to be monozygotic and monoamniotic a Caesarean section should be advised.
- Growth of babies should be assessed regularly to detect twin to twin transfusion and intrauterine growth retardation.

Advise epidural analgesia

If the presentation of the twins is anything other than vertex–vertex, this can be justified in terms of analgesia for possible intrauterine manipulations required in the second stage for delivery of the second twin. A satisfactory alternative is to have an anaesthetist present to administer an anaesthetic if complications arise.

Syntocinon should be available for the second stage

If contractions do not ensue within 5–10 minutes after delivery of the first twin, then an oxytocin infusion should be started.

Confirm the lie of the second twin, with ultrasound if necessary

If the lie is longitudinal with a cephalic presentation, wait until the head is descending and then perform amniotomy with a contraction.

If the lie of the second twin is transverse attempt external cephalic version without delay

This is to correct the lie to cephalic or breech.

If external cephalic version is unsuccessful either carry out internal podalic version and breech extraction or perform a Caesarean section

Internal podalic version

A fetal foot is identified by recognizing a heel through intact membranes. The foot is grasped and pulled gently and continuously lower into the birth canal. The membranes are ruptured as late as possible. The baby is then delivered as an assisted breech or breech extraction with pelvifemoral traction Lovset's manoeuvre to the shoulders and a controlled delivery of the head. This procedure is easiest when the transverse lie is with the back superior or posterior. If the back is inferior or if the limbs are not immediately palpable, ultrasound may help to identify where they would be found. This will minimize the risk of the unwanted experience of bringing down a fetal hand and arm in the mistaken belief that it is a foot.

Carry out assisted delivery of the second twin if there is a delay. The ventouse is preferred if the fetus presents cephalically

The ventouse has the advantages that it may be applied at a higher station than the forceps and causes less vaginal or perineal trauma. If the cervix is no longer fully dilated, using a 4 cm cup may be easier. The operator must be experienced.

Locked twins are very uncommon and are delivered by Caesarean section, as are the even rarer conjoined twins

Many clinicians choose Caesarean section when the first twin presents as a breech because of concern about 'interlocking' but this complication is extremely rare.

SYSTEMATIC REVIEW

Crowther CA (1999) Caesarean delivery for the second twin (Cochrane Review). *The Cochrane Library*, Issue 2. Update Software, Oxford.

Reviewers' conclusions: *Caesarean section delivery of a second twin not presenting cephalically is associated with increased maternal febrile morbidity with, as yet, no identified improvement in neonatal outcome. This policy should not be adopted except within the context of further controlled trials.*

USEFUL TELEPHONE NUMBER

Twins and Multiple Births Association (TAMBA)   01732 868000

UTERINE RUPTURE

E. O'Donnell and C. Cox

Ruptured uterus is a relatively rare event complicating 0.3/1000 deliveries. Prompt diagnosis and treatment are crucial if the baby is to be saved. Prolonged delays in diagnosis may lead to maternal mortality.

ACTION PLAN

1 **Suspect – beware of fetal distress in association with a risk factor for uterine rupture**

2 **Airway**
- Assess.
- Maintain patency.
- Apply oxygen 15 l/min via tight fitting face mask with reservoir bag.
- Attach pulse oximeter to patient.
- Call anaesthetist.
- Consider tracheal intubation.

Breathing
- Assess.
- Ventilate.
- Protect airway.

Circulation
- Assess pulse and BP.
- CPR if necessary.
- Put on ECG and automatic BP monitor.
- Treat peri-arrest arrhythmias.
- Secure i.v. access using two large bore cannulae.
- Send bloods for FBC, cross-match 6 units and clotting screen.
- Replace intravascular volume as necessary.

3 **Call senior obstetrician**

4 **If baby alive, head fully engaged and the cervix fully dilated a vaginal instrumental delivery may be carried out**

5 **Obtain consent for laparotomy and hysterectomy**

6 **Perform an urgent laparotomy under general anaesthesia administered by an experienced anaesthetist**

7 **The type of operation performed is dictated by the size and site of rupture, the degree of haemorrhage and the patient's future fertility wishes**

8 **Give prophylactic antibiotics**

9 **Document fully in notes, incident, assessment, treatments and management plan with date, time a signature and printed identification**

CONSULT OTHER TOPICS

Airway obstruction (p. 1)
Caesarean hysterectomy (p. 52)
Cardiopulmonary resuscitation (p. 8)
Hypotension (p. 150)
Instrumental delivery – forceps (p. 75)
Instrumental delivery – ventouse (p. 78)
Jehovah's Witness patient (p. 153)
Massive obstetric haemorrhage – antepartum (p. 88)
Massive obstetric haemorrhage – postpartum (p. 95)
Neonatal resuscitation (p. 14)
Peri-arrest arrhythmias (p. 16)
Respiratory emergencies (p. 20)

SUPPLEMENTARY INFORMATION

Suspect – beware of fetal distress in association with a risk factor for uterine rupture

- Commonest sign is prolonged fetal heart deceleration (in 70%).
- Other signs are pain and bleeding, both of which are unreliable (in only 7.6% and 3.4%, respectively).
- Cessation of uterine contractions associated with cardiotocographic evidence of fetal distress is particularly suggestive of uterine rupture.
- Pathological pain will usually come through an adequate epidural.

  Risk factors are

- previous Caesarean section especially associated with the use of oxytocic agents
- previous uterine trauma/surgery
- oxytocic usage in multiparous patients
- mullerian tract anomalies
- forceps deliveries, especially Kielland's forceps
- the multiparous woman who has delivered normally before and has a significantly bigger baby or a malposition in the present pregnancy and is allowed a prolonged second stage in the belief that she will deliver soon

The type of operation performed is dictated by the size and site of rupture, the degree of haemorrhage, and the patient's future fertility wishes

Dehiscence of the lower uterine segment in association with a previous Caesarean section is the most common operative finding.

- The rupture may extend anteriorly towards the back of the bladder, laterally towards the uterine arteries, or into the broad ligament plexus of veins and thereby lead to massive haemorrhage.
- Posterior rupture may occur and is usually associated with intrauterine malformations but has occurred in patients who have had a previous caesarean section and an obstructed labour and also after rotational forceps delivery.
- Sustained haemorrhage is an indication for performing a total or subtotal hysterectomy. Subtotal hysterectomy is a simpler procedure than total hysterectomy and reduces the risk of damage to the bladder and ureter.

Uterine Rupture

- Total hysterectomy may be performed, depending on the experience of the operator and the condition of the patient. The prime consideration is to preserve the patient's life.

REFERENCES

Farmer RM, Kirschbaum T and Potter D (1991) Uterine rupture during trial of labour after previous cesarean section. *Am. J. Obstet. Gynecol.* **165(4)**: 996–1001.

Fedorkow DM, Nimrod CA and Taylor PJ (1987) Ruptured uterus in pregnancy: A Canadian hospitals experience. *Can. Med. Assoc. J.* **137**: 27–29.

Gardeil F, Daly S and Turner MJ (1994) Uterine rupture and pregnancy reviewed. *Eur. J. Obstet. Gynecol. Reprod. Biol.* **56(2)**: 107–110.

ACUTE CHEST PAIN

The importance in treating chest pain is to make an early diagnosis of the life-threatening causes and to manage them accordingly. Chest pain is usually unrelated to pregnancy but may be exacerbated by it, e.g. heartburn from gastro-intestinal reflux or musculoskeletal pain.

1 **Airway**
- Assess.
- Maintain patency.
- Apply oxygen 15 l/min via tight fitting face mask with reservoir bag.
- Attach pulse oximeter to patient.
- Call anaesthetist.

Breathing
- Assess.
- Ventilate.
- Protect airway.

Circulation
- Assess.
- CPR.
- Put on ECG and automatic NIBP monitor.
- Treat peri-arrest arrhythmias.
- i.v. access, send bloods for FBC, U&Es, cardiac enzymes, G&S or cross-match, start i.v.i.
- Treat hypotension.

2 **Assess cause of pain and treat specifically**

3 **Exclude tension pneumothorax**
- Decompress immediately if clinical signs.

4 **Call for other specialty help (physicians, thoracic or general surgeons) in assessment and treatment**

5 **Arrange CXR and ECG and send arterial blood gases**

6 **Continuously monitor fetal heart by cardiotocography and consider timing and method of delivery**

7 **Keep record chart of pulse, BP, RR, SaO$_2$, temperature, FH and treatments given**

8 **Consider transfer to CCU or ICU**

9 **Record examination, investigations and diagnosis in notes and inform consultant obstetrician if appropriate**

CONSULT OTHER TOPICS

Acute abdominal pain (p. 44)
Airway obstruction (p. 1)
Cardiopulmonary resuscitation (p. 8)
Hypotension (p. 150)
Peri-arrest arrhythmias (p. 16)
Respiratory emergencies (p. 20)
Risk management (p. 185)

SUPPLEMENTARY INFORMATION

Assess cause of pain and treat specifically

Causes a–d are life-threatening.

(a) Myocardial infarction.
(b) Pulmonary embolus.
(c) Aortic dissection.
(d) Tension or simple pneumothorax.
(e) Pleurisy.
(f) Pneumonia.
(g) Pericarditis.
(h) Abdominal pain.
(i) Musculoskeletal pain.

Myocardial infarction pain is central, crushing and may radiate to the arms, jaw or upper abdomen. It is associated with dyspnoea and nausea and vomiting. Signs include clamminess, pulmonary oedema, cardiac arrhythmias and hypotension. Diagnosis is confirmed by serial ECGs and changes in cardiac enzyme levels.

A major pulmonary embolus may cause cardiovascular collapse. Pain from pulmonary emboli is pleuritic. Signs include a mild pyrexia, pleural rub, dyspnoea, cyanosis, tachycardia, hypotension and a raised JVP. There may be right axis deviation on the ECG and diagnosis is confirmed by Ventilation/Perfusion (V/Q) scan.

Aortic dissection presents as sudden onset of a tearing pain, retrosternally or in the back. There may be an absent pulse in one of the arms, a difference of blood pressure in the arms, a pericardial or pleural rub, hypotension, tachycardia, raised JVP and altered consciousness or weakness.

A pneumothorax causes pleuritic chest pain.

Pleurisy, pneumonia and pericarditis present as pleuritic pain.

Exclude tension pneumothorax

A tension pneumothorax must be quickly diagnosed and treated. It causes deviation of the trachea away from the affected side, reduced expansion on the affected side, hyperresonant percussion note on the affected side, reduced breath sounds on the affected side, hypotension, tachycardia and raised JVP. It must be decompressed immediately by inserting a cannula into the second intercostal space at the midclavicular line. A chest drain must be inserted subsequently.

ACUTE SEVERE ASTHMA

Asthma is caused by bronchospasm and is usually recognized by a wheeze.

Signs of severe asthma are inability to complete sentences in one breath, RR > 25 breaths/min, HR greater than 110/min, use of accessory muscles of respiration and a peak expiratory flow of < 50% predicted (predicted = 480 l/min).

Signs of life-threatening asthma are a silent chest, cyanosis or feeble respiratory effort, exhaustion, confusion, coma, bradycardia or hypotension and a peak expiratory flow of < 33% predicted (approx 160 l/min).

The peak expiratory flow rate (PEFR) can be measured at the bedside by asking the patient to exhale forcefully into a peak flow meter.

ACTION PLAN

1 **Call for help including resident anaesthetist, obstetrician and medical registrar**

2 **Give humidified oxygen 40–60%**

3 **Give salbutamol**
   - 5 mg in 3 ml normal saline as nebulizer via oxygen mask.

4 **Secure venous access, send blood samples for FBC, U&Es, blood glucose and start i.v. fluids 1 l normal saline, 8 hourly**

5 **Give hydrocortisone 200 mg i.v.**

6 **Attach pulse oximeter to the patient**
   - If SaO_2 < 92% or patient has any life-threatening features, measure arterial blood gases.

7 **Put on NIBP and ECG monitor**

8 **Check medical registrar has been summoned**

9 **Repeat PEFR measurement every 15 min**

10 **Repeat salbutamol 5 mg via nebulizer up to every 15 min until improvement**

11 **If life-threatening attack or not improving after 15 min**
   - Add ipratropium 500 µg to a repeat dose of salbutamol 5 mg via nebulizer.
   - Give i.v. aminophylline 250 µg over 10 min under ECG control.

12 **Exclude tension pneumothorax; decompress if there is one**

13 **Be prepared to intubate if deteriorating PEFR, persisting PaO_2 of < 8 kPa, deteriorating PaO_2, $PaCO_2$ of > 4 kPa, exhaustion or drowsiness**
   - Call anaesthetist.

14 **Organize portable CXR to exclude pneumothorax or consolidation**

15 **Send arterial blood gases**

Acute Severe Asthma

16 **Check fetal heart and continuously monitor by cardiotoco-graphy – consider timing and method of delivery**

17 **Consider cause of bronchospasm**

18 **Keep record chart of pulse, BP, RR, SaO$_2$, FH and drugs given**

19 **Record in notes and inform consultant obstetrician**

CONSULT OTHER TOPICS

Anaphylaxis (p. 133)
Cardiopulmonary resuscitation (p. 8)
Hypotension (p. 150)
Peri-arrest arrhythmias (p. 16)
Respiratory emergencies (p. 20)

SUPPLEMENTARY INFORMATION

Give humidified oxygen 40–60%

CO_2 retention is not aggravated by oxygen therapy in asthma.

Give salbutamol

This may have the predicted β2 sympathomimetic effect of relaxing uterine muscle. However, severe bronchospasm is life-threatening to mother and fetus and should be treated with this conventional therapy.

Give hydrocortisone 200 mg i.v.

Repeat 4-hourly if necessary.

Repeat PEFR measurement every 15 min

Improvement is signified by a rise in peak expiratory flow to above 50% predicted.

If life-threatening attack or not improving after 15 min

- Add ipratropium 500 µg to a repeat dose of salbutamol 5 mg via nebulizer. Ipratropium may cause urinary retention.
- Give i.v. aminophyline 250 µg over 10 min under ECG control.
  Although theophyllines have been given in late pregnancy without adverse effect there are reports of neonatal irritability and apnoea. If aminophylline is given therefore the resident paediatrician should be informed. Aminophylline should not be given to patients already taking oral theophyllines.

Exclude tension pneumothorax

Signs of a tension pneumothorax include deviation of the trachea away from the affected side, reduced expansion of the chest on the affected side, hyperresonant

Acute Severe Asthma

percussion note on the affected side, reduced air entry on the affected side, tachycardia and hypotension.

The tension pneumothorax can be relieved in an emergency situation by inserting an intravenous cannula into the second intercostal space in the mid-clavicular line on the affected side. A chest drain must be placed subsequently.

Send arterial blood gases

A $PaCO_2$ of > 4 kPa or a PaO_2 of < 8 kPa are signs of severe respiratory compromise.

REFERENCE

British Thoracic Society (1993) Guidelines for the management of asthma: a summary. *Br. Med. J.* **306**: 776–782.

ANAPHYLAXIS

Anaphylaxis is an exaggerated response to a substance to which an individual has become sensitized, in which histamine, serotonin and other vasoactive substances are released. This causes symptoms which can include pruritus, erythema, flushing, urticaria, angio-oedema, nausea, diarrhoea, vomiting, laryngeal oedema, bronchospasm, hypotension, cardiovascular collapse and death. Anaphylactic reactions usually begin within 5–10 min of exposure and the full reaction usually evolves within 30 min. Anaphylactic and anaphylactoid reactions are indistinguishable and managed in the same way. They have a different immunological mechanism. In a patient with latex allergy repeated vaginal examination with gloves containing latex and other exposure to latex can lead to anaphylaxis.

ACTION PLAN

1 **Diagnosis is made on clinical grounds – suspect**

2 **Stop administration of drug(s)/blood product likely to have caused anaphylaxis**

3 **Call for help including anaesthetist**

4 **Airway**
- Assess.
- Maintain patency.
- Apply oxygen 15 l/min via tight fitting face mask with reservoir bag.
- Attach pulse oximeter to patient.
- Consider tracheal intubation.

Breathing
- Assess.
- Ventilate.
- Protect airway.

Circulation
- Assess pulse, BP.
- CPR.
- Tilt to left.
- Put on ECG and BP monitor.
- Treat peri-arrest arrhythmias.
- Secure i.v. access with large bore cannula.

5 **Lie patient in left lateral tilt, head down**

6 **Give adrenaline/epinephrine**
- *Either* 0.5 mg to 1 mg (0.5 to 1 ml of 1:1000) intramuscularly every 10 min until improvement in pulse and blood pressure.
- *Or* 50 to 100 µg (0.5 to 1 ml of 1:10 000) i.v. titrated against blood pressure.
- If cardiovascular collapse 0.5 to 1 mg (5 to 10 ml of 1:10 000) may be required i.v. in divided doses titrated against response.

Give at a rate of 0.1 mg/min and stop when a response has been obtained.

7 **Start intravascular volume expansion with crystalloid or synthetic colloid**

8 **Give secondary therapy**
- Antihistamines: chlorpheniramine 10–20 mg by slow i.v. infusion. Consider ranitidine 50 mg i.v.
- Corticosteroids: hydrocortisone 100–300 mg i.v.

9 **Reassess airway, breathing and circulation**

10 **Consider catecholamines if blood pressure still low**
- Adrenaline/epinephrine 0.05–0.1 µg/kg/min (approx 4–8 µg/min) 5 mg adrenaline/epinephrine in 500 ml saline gives 10 µg/ml.
- Noradrenaline/norepinephrine 0.05–0.1 µg/kg/min (approx 4–8 µg/min) 4 mg noradrenaline/norepinephrine in 500 ml dextrose gives 8 µg/ml.

11 **Perform arterial blood gases**
- Consider bicarbonate for acidosis (0.5–1.0 mmol/kg i.v.). 0.5–1.0 mmol is equivalent to 0.5–1.0 ml of an 8.4% solution of sodium bicarbonate.

12 **Consider bronchodilators if persistent bronchospasm**
- e.g. salbutamol 2.5 mg via oxygen driven nebulizer or 250 µg i.v. slowly.
- *Or* aminophylline 250 mg i.v. over 20 min.

13 **Check fetal heart and continuously monitor by cardiotocography and consider timing and method of delivery**

14 **Keep a record chart to include pulse, BP, RR, SaO$_2$, FH and treatments given**

15 **Document in notes with time, date, a signature and printed identification and inform consultant obstetrician**

16 **Investigate**

CONSULT OTHER TOPICS

Anaphylaxis

SUPPLEMENTARY INFORMATION

Diagnosis is made on clinical grounds – suspect

The diagnosis is likely if flushing and urticaria, wheezing and hypotension coexist. Consider as a cause of cardiac arrest.

Clinical Features	Frequency (%)
Cardiovascular collapse	88
Bronchospasm	36
Angio-oedema	24
(face, periorbital, perioral)	
Generalized oedema	7
Cutaneous signs:	
rash	13
erythema	45
urticaria	8.5
First clinical feature	
No pulse, low BP	28
Flushing	26
Coughing	6
Rash	4
Cyanosis	3
Others (urticaria, swelling)	9

Stop administration of drug(s)/blood product likely to have caused anaphylaxis

As the cause, suspect any drug, infusion or blood or blood product currently being administered or given in the last 30 min. Anaphylactic reactions are more common when drugs are given intravenously.

Document in notes with time, date, a signature and printed identification and inform consultant obstetrician

The doctor who administered/prescribed the drug/infusion/blood should ensure that the reaction is recorded appropriately in the notes. It is important to document timing of administration of all drugs in relation to onset of reaction. The responsible consultant should be informed immediately. The patient's General Practitioner must be notified. The patient should be given advice on further investigation, an explanation of events and a written record of the reaction. All suspected anaphylactic drug reactions should be reported to the Committee on the Safety of Medicines.

Investigate

Consider possibility of coagulopathy. Approximately 1 hour after the beginning of the reaction 10 ml of venous blood should be taken in a glass tube. The serum should be separated and stored at $-20°C$ until it can be sent to a reference laboratory for serum tryptase concentration estimation which may be elevated in an anaphylactic reaction

Any patient who has had a suspected anaphylactic reaction should be investigated fully. This is best done by referring the patient to an allergy clinic. The investigation should be conducted in consultation with an allergist or clinical immunologist. No blood test identifies the causative agent but other tests should be introduced on the advice of the allergist. Skin testing, radioallergosorbent testing (RAST) for specific drugs, or latex agglutination testing may be recommended. The British Society of Allergy and Immunology publishes a list of members able to advise.

LATEX PROTEIN ALLERGY

In care of these patients latex should be avoided:

- Identify products containing latex and provide a list of alternatives.
- Ensure alternatives available and accessible at all times and kept in a specified place.
- Every member of staff having direct physical contact with the patient should ensure that whatever they wear or use does not contain latex.

The following products/equipment should not be used; latex-containing gloves, Foley's in-dwelling catheters, blood i.v. sets with rubber injection site, Luer lock caps, rubber face masks, Entonox rubber tubing, elasticated straps for use with CTG monitor, tourniquets, rubber mattress covers on theatre tables, beds, wedges, trolleys, etc., sphygmomanometer tubing, elastoplast, multidose bottles with rubber stopper, e.g. lignocaine bottles.

REFERENCES

The Association of Anaesthetists of Great Britain and Ireland and The British Society of Allergy and Clinical Immunology (1995) *Suspected Anaphylactic Reactions Associated with Anaesthesia*, revised edition. Association of Anaesthetists, London.
Ewan PW (1998) ABC of Allergies: Anaphylaxis. *Br. Med. J.* **316**: 1442–1445.

CONFUSION

Confusion is usually implied by irrational opinion or behaviour. Intrapartum, attention must be paid to its cause, the difficulties encountered in obstetric care of a confused patient and the problems in obtaining consent for treatment or refusal of treatment.

ACTION PLAN

1 **Take history, examine and investigate to find cause and treat if applicable**

2 **If evidence of psychiatric illness take advice from psychiatrists**

3 **Give explanation and reassurance to patient**

4 **Consider issues of consent**

5 **Call consultant obstetrician who will decide what is in the best interest of the patient by balancing the need and risk. Consider telephone advice from his/her medical defence organization**

6 **Document, in full, decisions to give treatment against patient's will or where treatment has been carried out without consent with time, date, a signature and printed identification**

7 **Retrospectively assess cause and follow-up**

CONSULT OTHER TOPICS

Airway obstruction (p. 1)
Consent (p. 183)
Diabetic emergencies – diabetic ketoacidosis (p. 139)
Diabetic emergencies – hypoglycaemia (p. 142)
Respiratory emergencies (p. 20)
Risk management (p. 185)

SUPPLEMENTARY INFORMATION

Take history, examine and investigate to find cause. Treat if applicable

- Hypoxia.
- Hypotension.
- Sepsis.
- Drugs or drug withdrawal.
- Metabolic causes especially hypoglycaemia.
- Cerebral causes, especially pre-eclampsia.

Confusion

- Endocrine causes.
- Permanent mental disability.
- Psychiatric illness.

If evidence of psychiatric illness take advice from psychiatrists

Improving the psychiatric illness may make the labour more manageable. Psychiatrist will consider whether a Treatment Order should be issued according to the Mental Health Act 1983. Note that even if the patient is sectioned under the Mental Health Act treatment can only be enforced for her *psychiatric* condition.

Give explanation and reassurance to patient

Try to address her anxieties. Attempt to 'talk down' an aggressive patient and avoid confrontation.

Consider issues of consent

It must be decided whether the patient is capable of giving consent. This depends on her capacity to make an informed decision.

In the case of adults who are incapable of giving a valid consent, no parent, guardian or court has the power to consent on behalf of the patient. The issue of giving treatment to incompetent adults was addressed by the House of Lords in the case of F v *West Berkshire Health Authority*.The law lords confirmed that no one could consent on behalf of an incompetent adult but that it would be intolerable for adult incompetent patients to be denied treatment on the grounds that a consent could not be obtained. In these circumstances they said that doctors should act to protect the best interests of their patients by treating them in accordance with a responsible body of medical opinion.

If patients comply you may carry out investigations or treatments which you believe to be in their best interests. If they do not comply they can only be *compulsorily* treated for their *mental disorder* or a physical disorder arising from the mental disorder.

The 1983 Mental Health Act provides the legal basis for compulsory admission, detention and treatment.

REFERENCE

General Medical Council. Seeking patients' consent: the ethical considerations.

USEFUL TELEPHONE NUMBERS

Medical Defence Union	0171 935 5503
	0161 491 3301
Medical Protection Society	0171 399 1300
	0113 243 6436
Medical and Dental Defence Union of Scotland	0141 221 5858

Confusion

DIABETIC EMERGENCIES – DIABETIC KETOACIDOSIS

Loss of consciousness due to hypoglycaemia is of rapid onset. A reduced level of consciousness due to diabetic ketoacidosis (DKA) is of more gradual onset. BMstix and laboratory blood glucose levels distinguish the two. Hypoglycaemia is immediately life-threatening, therefore if in doubt give 50 ml i.v. dextrose 50%. Babies of diabetic mothers, particularly mothers who require emergency management of their diabetes, are at risk of neonatal hypoglycaemia.

1 **Suspect**

2 **Airway**
- Assess.
- Maintain patency.
- Apply oxygen 15 l/min via tight fitting face mask with reservoir bag.
- Attach pulse oximeter.
- Call anaesthetist.

Breathing
- Assess.
- Ventilate.
- Protect airway.

Circulation
- Assess pulse and BP.
- CPR.
- Tilt to left.
- Put on ECG monitor.
- Treat peri-arrest arrhythmias.
- I.v. access, send bloods for blood glucose, U&Es, FBC, start i.v.i. 5% dextrose.
- Treat hypotension.

3 **The principles of further treatment are rehydration, correction of electrolyte imbalance, treatment of hyperglycaemia**

4 **Call diabetic team/physicians. There may be guidelines in place locally. This is a complex condition and requires specialist management**

5 **Continuously monitor fetal heart by cardiotocography and consider timing and method of delivery**

6 **Catheterize, check urine for ketones to confirm diagnosis and measure urine output every 15 minutes**

7 **Send arterial blood gases and blood cultures**

8 **Rehydrate**

9 **Give insulin**

10 **Add potassium to i.v. fluid when the potassium level is known**

11 **Repeat blood glucose, U&Es and arterial blood gases**

12 **Keep a record chart to include pulse, BP, RR, SaO$_2$, blood glucose measurements, potassium levels, blood gases, FH and treatments given**

13 **Document event and treatment in notes, with time, date, a signature and printed identification and inform consultant obstetrician**

CONSULT OTHER TOPICS

Airway obstruction (p. 1)
Cardiopulmonary resuscitation (p. 8)
Confusion (p. 137)
Loss of consciousness or fitting (p. 157)
Respiratory emergencies (p. 20)
Shoulder dystocia (p. 119)

SUPPLEMENTARY INFORMATION

Suspect

In an unconscious, insulin-dependent diabetic – based on clinical features. Biochemical definition blood glucose > 9 mmol/l (can occur at much lower levels however) ketonuria 1:2 or greater and metabolic acidosis, or in a known insulin-dependent diabetic with infection, trauma or reason for inadequate insulin intake. There has usually been gradual onset of polyuria and drowsiness. The patient is dry, tachypnoeic, hypotensive, taking deep sighing respirations and smells of ketones. DKA can be the presentation of diabetes.

The principles of further treatment are rehydration, correction of electrolyte imbalance, treatment of hyperglycaemia

Metabolic acidosis corrects as the other physiological variables return to normal. Physicians may choose to treat it, but this should be a decision left to the experts.

Continuously monitor fetal heart by cardiotocography and consider timing and method of delivery

The fetus is at significant risk for sudden intrauterine death during an episode of diabetic ketoacidosis. Monitor fetus carefully. Delivery of a compromised baby should be cautiously delayed until the mother is metabolically stable. Correction of maternal metabolic abnormalities improves the fetus's condition. Emergency operative intervention should be reserved for unresponsive fetal compromise. Inform paediatrician and SCBU. Mother may require high dependency facilities-these may need to be provided on the delivery suite depending on obstetric needs.

Send arterial blood gases and blood cultures

There may be a metabolic acidosis and treatment of this should be discussed with anaesthetist/diabetic physician. An infective cause of DKA is sought.

Rehydrate

With normal saline 500 ml stat followed by 1000 ml over the next hour if the diagnosis is confirmed. Continue resuscitation with normal saline until blood glucose < 11 mmol/l and then replace with dextrose saline. Consider CVP line.

Give insulin

Actrapid insulin 0.1 units/kg i.v. stat and make up insulin infusion by adding 50 units to 500 ml normal salute (0.1 unit/ml) and run at 0.1 unit/kg/hour (1 ml/ kg/hour).

Add potassium to i.v. fluid when the potassium level is known

If K:	Give:
< 3.0 mmol/l	40 mmol (3 g) KCl/hour
3.0–4.0 mmol/l	26.8 mmol (2 g) KCl/hour
4.0–5.0 mmol/l	20 mmol (1.5 g) KCl/hour
5.0–6.0 mmol/l	13.4 mmol (1 g) KCl/hour

Stop potassium if patient is anuric, level > 6.0 mmol/l or ECG shows peaked T waves or widening of QRS complex.

For guidelines for the control of blood glucose during labour in insulin-treated women, see Appendix I, p. 187.

REFERENCE

Foley MR and Strong TH (1997) Diabetic ketoacidosis in pregnancy. In: *Obstetric Intensive Care: a practical manual.* WB Saunders Company, Philadelphia.

DIABETIC EMERGENCIES –
HYPOGLYCAEMIA

Loss of consciousness due to hypoglycaemia is of rapid onset. A reduced level of consciousness due to diabetic ketoacidosis is of more gradual onset. BMstix and laboratory blood glucose levels distinguish the two. Hypoglycaemia is immediately life-threatening, therefore if in doubt give 50 ml i.v. dextrose 50%. Babies of diabetic mothers, particularly mothers who require emergency management of their diabetes, are at risk of neonatal hypoglycaemia.

1 **Airway**
   - Assess.
   - Maintain patency.
   - Apply oxygen 15 l/min via tight fitting face mask with reservoir bag.
   - Attach pulse oximeter.
   - Call anaesthetist.

   Breathing
   - Assess.
   - Ventilate.
   - Protect airway.

   Circulation
   - Assess pulse and BP.
   - CPR.
   - Tilt to left.
   - Put on ECG monitor.
   - Treat peri-arrest arrhythmias.
   - i.v. access, send bloods for blood glucose, U&Es, FBC, start i.v.i. 5% dextrose.
   - Treat hypotension.

2 **If 'BMstix' show glucose of < 2.3 mmol/l treatment should be given without waiting for a laboratory blood glucose result**

3 **Give 50 ml of 50% dextrose i.v.**

4 **Glucagon 1 mg i.m. may be given if the i.v. route is unavailable**

5 **When consciousness is restored consider cause**

6 **Blood sugar as by BMstix should be between 4 and 9 mmol/l. Check BMstix every 30 min. Start GKI (glucose, potassium, insulin) regimen (see below)**

7 **Call diabetic physicians for further management**

8 **Continuously monitor fetal heart by cardiotocography and consider timing and method of delivery**

9 Keep a record to include pulse, BP, RR, SaO$_2$, BMstix reading, FH and treatments given

10 Document event and treatment in notes, with time, date, a signature and printed identification and inform consultant obstetrician

CONSULT OTHER TOPICS

Airway obstruction (p. 1)
Cardiopulmonary resuscitation (p. 8)
Confusion (p. 137)
Loss of consciousness or fitting (p. 157)
Respiratory emergencies (p. 20)
Shoulder dystocia (p. 119)

SUPPLEMENTARY INFORMATION

When consciousness is restored consider cause

Patients who have taken long-acting insulins or very large doses of insulin may require 10% dextrose drip for 24–48 hours to stop hypoglycaemia recurring.

Continuously monitor fetal heart by cardiotocography and consider timing and method of delivery

Babies of diabetic mothers are at risk from neonatal hypoglycaemia. Symptomatic hypoglycaemia results in handicap in up to 50%. Inform paediatrician and SCBU.

For guidelines for the control of blood glucose during labour in insulin-treated women, see Appendix I, p. 187.

HIV AND AIDS

HIV can be diagnosed or undiagnosed.

ACTION PLAN

1 **Consider antenatal screening if at risk of HIV**

2 **Prevent vertical transmission**
   - Consider risk factors.
   - Advise Caesarean section.
   - Give zidovudine (AZT).
   - Advise against breastfeeding.

3 **Protect the professional**

4 **Refer to HIV physician and for counselling when diagnosed**

5 **Discuss case antenatally with paediatrician**

6 **Attend to issues of risk management**

CONSULT OTHER TOPICS

Puerperal sepsis, septicaemia and septic shock (p. 113)
Risk management (p. 185)
Substance abuse (p. 173)

SUPPLEMENTARY INFORMATION

Prevent vertical transmission

Vertical transmission accounts for 85% of all paediatric infections – 15% in the UK and USA; 45% in sub-Saharan Africa.
   It can occur

- Antenatally (in utero).
- Intrapartum (at delivery) – probably accounts for the majority of cases.
- Postpartum (breastfeeding).

Consider risk factors

- Advanced maternal disease.
- High maternal viral load.
- Immunosuppression.
- Prolonged rupture of the membranes.
- Vaginal delivery.
- Prematurity.
- Breastfeeding.
- Invasive procedures, e.g. chorionic villus sampling, amniocentesis, fetal blood sampling and internal monitoring.

Associated risk factors

- Unprotected sexual intercourse during pregnancy.
- Use of illicit drugs.
- Cigarette smoking.
- Non-use of zidovudine (AZT).

Advise Caesarean section

Reduces vertical transmission by reducing fetal contact with potentially infectious material.

Give zidovudine

- Reduces vertical transmission by 70%.
- Using antiretroviral drugs (e.g. nevirapine) in addition to Caesarean section may reduce rate of vertical transmission to 1%.

Protect the professional

- The majority of women who have HIV are unaware as they have not been tested and may only become aware when the baby develops an illness such as pneumocystis carinii pneumonia.
- In pregnancy, abortion and delivery, body fluids may be shed in large amounts, often unexpectedly.
- Lochia is normal after childbirth.
- There is a small but established risk of transmission through cuts, abrasions or mucous membranes.

If there is a definite risk of infection the following steps should be carried out:

- The delivery team should be kept to a minimum.
- Staff with skin conditions such as eczema should not be involved.
- Cuts and abrasions must be covered with waterproof dressings.
- Staff should wear a plastic apron under their gowns.
- Waterproof footwear and gloves should be worn.
- Eye protection should be worn.
- Vaginal examinations should be kept to a minimum.

For delivery:

- Scalp electrodes and fetal blood sampling should be avoided.
- Forceps may be preferable to the ventouse for assisted delivery.
- Manual removal of the placenta requires surgical gauntlets.
- Contamination should be dealt with by sodium hypochlorite containing 10 000 p.p.m. available chlorine.

If inoculation is thought to have occurred, immediate contact should be made with the infection control, sister or microbiologist with a view to the administration of prophylactic antiviral therapy.

Refer to HIV physician and for counselling when diagnosed

When diagnosis is made refer to paediatrician for ongoing care or if clinical suspicion of AIDS.

Attend to issues of risk management

The names of all staff involved should be recorded.

SYSTEMATIC REVIEW

Brocklehurst P (1999) Interventions for reducing mother-to-child transmission of HIV infection (Cochrane Review). *The Cochrane Library*, Issue 2. Update Software, Oxford.

Reviewers' conclusions: *Zidovudine therapy appears to be very effective in decreasing the risk of mother-to-child transmission of HIV infection.*

HYPERTENSION

S. Maguire and K. Grady

The 1994–1996 Report on Confidential Enquiries into Maternal Deaths in the United Kingdom found pregnancy induced hypertension (PIH) to be the second leading cause of direct death.

The aetiology of hypertension in pregnancy is

(a) Chronic hypertension which either predates pregnancy or develops before 20 weeks' gestation and is defined as BP > 140/90.
(b) Pregnancy induced hypertension which develops after 20 weeks' gestation in a normotensive woman.
(c) Gestational hypertension which is PIH in isolation, but may develop to pre-eclampsia.

The following action plan can be applied to any hypertensive patient, including the pre-eclamptic. Other aspects of the treatment of pre-eclampsia are covered in the dedicated chapter.

ACTION PLAN

1 **Seek advice from senior obstetrician. There may be local guidelines**

2 **If pre-eclamptic attend to other aspects of illness**

3 **Closely monitor fetus and consider timing and method of delivery**

4 **Treat severe hypertension in an area with invasive monitoring facilities**

5 **Secure i.v. access and send bloods for FBC, clotting studies, U&Es, LFTs and urate levels**

6 **Send urine for 24-hour urinary protein level and monitor urine output (no need to catheterize)**

7 **Commence antihypertensive medication if diastolic BP > 105**

8 **Choose antihypertensive depending on the experience and familiarity of an individual clinician with a particular drug**

9 **If blood pressure does not respond to the above discuss with senior renal physicians and senior anaesthetists who will supervise further treatment**

10 **Consider epidural analgesia to control blood pressure**

11 **Give plasma volume expanders**

12 **Examine for signs of left ventricular failure and arrange CXR**

13 **Keep record chart of pulse, BP, SaO_2, fluid intake, urine output, FH and treatments given**

14 **Postpartum, continue antihypertensives if diastolic > 110 mmHg or mean arterial pressure > 140 mmHg**

15 Record decisions and management plans in notes with times, date, a signature and printed identification

CONSULT OTHER TOPICS

Eclampsia, pre-eclampsia, HELLP, fatty liver and hepatic rupture (p. 66)
Loss of consciousness or fitting (p. 157)

SUPPLEMENTARY INFORMATION

If pre-eclamptic attend to other aspects of illness

Essential hypertension is a major predisposing factor for pre-eclampsia (increases risk 5-fold).

Treat severe hypertension in an area with invasive monitoring facilities

Regular NIBP and ECG monitoring is necessary and consider intra-arterial blood pressure monitoring if BP unstable.

Choose antihypertensive depending on the experience and familiarity of an individual clinician with a particular drug

Nifedipine 10 mg orally or sublingually with 300 ml of synthetic colloid to avoid precipitous fall in BP is suggested and can be repeated every 30 minutes according to response. If precipitous fall in BP occurs, ephedrine in 3 mg increments should be given i.v. and titrated against BP. Maintenance can be given as a slow release preparation 10 mg b.d. increasing to 20 mg b.d. An interaction between nifedipine and magnesium sulphate has been reported to produce profound maternal muscle weakness, maternal hypotension and fetal distress. The risk is small but labetolol may be preferred if magnesium sulphate is being used.

Labetolol is given as an initial i.v. bolus of 5 mg titrated against blood pressure and repeated at 5 minute intervals up to a dose of 1 mg/kg. Labetolol can precipitate heart failure and its use must be closely observed.

Hydralazine is commonly used. If there is no great urgency, the mother should receive a pre-loading infusion of 400 ml of 4.5% human albumin given over 20 minutes. Give 5 mg i.v. slowly. The onset of antihypertensive effect may be delayed. Additional doses can be given to a maximum dose of 20 mg, but only at intervals of 20 minutes. The effect of a single dose may last up to 6 hours. If no lasting effect with boluses (assess over 20 minutes), consider an infusion at 2.0 mg/hour increasing by 0.5 mg/hour as required (2-20 mg/hour usually required).

It has been found that, compared with intravenous hydralazine, nifedipine and labetolol were associated with less maternal hypotension, fewer Caesarean sections, fewer placental abruptions and fewer low Apgar scores.

Antihypertensive treatment benefits the mother with mild (diastolic 90-99 mmHg) to moderate (diastolic 100-109 mmHg) hypertension but there is no clear choice of drug.

If blood pressure does not respond to the above discuss with senior renal physicians and senior anaesthetists who will supervise further treatment

Other options include an infusion of nitroglycerin at 10 µg/min or sodium nitroprusside infusion at 0.05–0.1 µg/kg/min.

Consider epidural analgesia to control blood pressure

It is only indicated if the patient is in labour and is contraindicated in the presence of a coagulopathy.

Give plasma volume expanders

Plasma volume expansion is necessary because in severe pre-eclampsia there is an increase in systemic vascular resistance. If this is reduced by anti-hypertensives, a precipitous fall in blood pressure can result. The ideal is to gently reduce the systemic vascular resistance and simultaneously expand the intravascular volume, thereby improving end organ blood flow.

SYSTEMATIC REVIEW

Duley L and Henderson-Smart DJ (1999) Drugs for rapid treatment of very high blood pressure during pregnancy (Cochrane Review). *The Cochrane Library*, Issue 2. Update Software, Oxford.

Reviewers' conclusions: *Until better evidence is available, the choice of anti-hypertensive should depend on the experience and familiarity of an individual clinician with a particular drug, and on what is known about adverse maternal and fetal side effects. Exceptions are diazoxide and ketanserin, which are probably not good choices.*

REFERENCES

Magee LA, Ornstein MP and von Dadelszen P (1999) Management of hypertension in pregnancy. *Br. Med. J.* **318**: 1332–1336.
Scientific Advisory Committee of the Royal College of Obstetricians and Gynaecologists (1999) *Management of Eclampsia*. RCOG, London. (Valid until November 1999.)

HYPOTENSION

S. Maguire and K. Grady

This is much less well defined than hypertension in pregnancy, but a fall in systolic pressure of greater than 20 mmHg or a fall in the mean arterial pressure of greater than 20% would suggest hypotension. During normal pregnancy, blood pressure will fall during the second trimester with an average systolic fall of 5 mmHg up to the 28th week.

The causes of hypotension may be broadly defined as hypovolaemia, obstruction to venous return (aortocaval compression), pooling of blood in the extremities therefore causing reduced venous return (effect of epidural/spinal, septic shock) and reduced myocardial contractility (myocardial infarction, tension pneumothorax).

ACTION PLAN

1 **Call for help including senior obstetrician and resident anaesthetist**

2 **Airway**
- Assess.
- Maintain patency.
- Apply oxygen 15 l/min via tight fitting face mask attached to reservoir bag.
- Attach pulse oximeter.

Breathing
- Assess, exclude or treat tension pneumothorax.
- Assist breathing by ventilation if necessary.
- Protect airway.
- Consider anaphylaxis.

3 **Consider cause**

4 **Place patient in left lateral position**

5 **Turn off epidural infusion**

6 **Check pulse, BP, put on automatic BP machine and record BP every 3 min, put on ECG monitor, secure i.v. access**

7 **Start CPR and treat peri-arrest arrhythmias as necessary. Treat bradycardia with atropine 0.3 mg increments i.v.**

8 **Place two large i.v. cannulae, send bloods for FBC, cross-match, clotting studies, cultures and save for drug screen**

9 **Infuse normal saline 500 ml stat. If haemorrhage (may be concealed, but tachycardia is suggestive of haemorrhage) continue infusion of crystalloid/synthetic colloid/blood/ blood products as for massive obstetric haemorrhage. Warm fluids**

10 **If no suggestion of haemorrhage consider boluses of ephedrine 3 mg i.v. titrated against BP**

11 **Continually reassess effect of action/treatment**

12 **Catheterize and measure urine output**

13 **If treatment ineffective consider CVP to assess cause**

14 **If sepsis is suspected give i.v. fluids and call anaesthetist for transfer to ICU**

15 **If trauma, the cause of hypotension is most likely haemorrhage. Consider neurogenic shock if unresponsive to adequate volume replacement. Call anaesthetist for transfer to ICU**

16 **Check fetal heart and consider method and timing of delivery**

17 **Keep record chart to include pulse, BP, RR, SaO$_2$, CVP, urine output, FH and treatments given**

18 **Record in notes and inform consultant obstetrician if appropriate**

19 **Document findings and treatments in notes with time, date, a signature and printed identification**

CONSULT OTHER TOPICS

Airway obstruction (p. 1)
Anaphylaxis (p. 133)
Cardiopulmonary resuscitation (p. 8)
Loss of consciousness or fitting (p. 157)
Massive obstetric haemorrhage – antepartum (p. 88)
Massive obstetric haemorrhage – postpartum (p. 95)
Peri-arrest arrhythmias (p. 16)
Puerperal sepsis, septicaemia and septic shock (p. 113)
Respiratory emergencies (p. 20)
Spinals and epidurals – high spinal anaesthesia (p. 169)
Spinals and epidurals – local anaesthetic toxicity (p. 171)
Trauma (p. 24)

SUPPLEMENTARY INFORMATION

Breathing

A tension pneumothorax is a life-threatening cause of hypotension. The most likely cause is trauma but should be considered in any patient with deviation of the trachea, hyperresonant percussion note (affected side) and reduced breath sounds (affected side). The trachea is deviated away from the affected side. Do not wait for CXR to confirm diagnosis. Decompress immediately by inserting a cannula through the second intercostal space in the midclavicular line on the affected side.

Consider cause

- Aortocaval compression.
- Anaphylaxis.

Hypotension

151

- Epidural or spinal.
- Hypovolaemia.
- Sepsis.
- Cardiac cause – vagally induced bradycardia, arrhythmias, myocardial infarction, cardiac tamponade.
- Respiratory cause – tension pneumothorax, pulmonary embolus.
- Illegal drug ingestion or drug overdose.
- Neurogenic shock in trauma.
- Septic patients who are hypotensive may have septic shock but other causes should first be excluded, e.g. aortocaval compression, hypovolaemia. CVP and possibly pulmonary artery pressure measurements are needed to make the diagnosis. Septic shock should be treated in ICU or HDU by judicious control of intravascular volume and ionotropes.

If no suggestion of haemorrhage consider boluses of ephedrine 3 mg i.v. titrated against BP

Conventionally ephedrine 30 mg is diluted to 10 ml and increments of 3 mg (1 ml) are titrated against response.

If trauma, the cause of hypotension is most likely haemorrhage – consider neurogenic shock if unresponsive to adequate volume replacement – call anaesthetist for transfer to ICU

The most likely cause of hypotension in the injured patient is haemorrhage. If intravascular replacement is adequate and the patient has persistent hypotension, without cutaneous vasoconstriction, tachycardia and without a rise in diastolic pressure, suspect neurogenic shock, caused by loss of sympathetic tone due to spinal cord injury.

SYSTEMATIC REVIEW

Offringa M (1998) Excess mortality after human albumin administration in critically ill patients. Clinical and pathophysiological evidence suggests albumin is harmful. *Br. Med. J.* **317**: 223–224.

JEHOVAH'S WITNESS PATIENT

The contents of this chapter have been approved by the Manchester Hospital Liaison Committee for Jehovah's Witnesses and by the Jehovah's Witnesses' Hospital Information Services Department.

For religious reasons, Jehovah's Witnesses believe that blood transfusion is forbidden. This is a deeply held core value and they regard a non-consensual transfusion as a gross physical violation. Witnesses view scripture as ruling out transfusion of whole blood, packed red blood cells, white blood cells, plasma, and platelets. Witnesses' religious understanding does not absolutely prohibit the use of minor blood fractions such as clotting factors. Jehovah's witnesses are not 'anti-medicine' and wish to be treated with effective non-blood medical alternatives to allogeneic blood. A doctor is obliged to give the best care to his patient in keeping with the patient's wishes. He should know of non-blood medical alternatives in advance and plan optimal care for each individual patient. Early knowledge of the patient's refusal of blood products is essential. This should be clearly documented and all members of the obstetric team should be made aware of the situation and of the care/contingency plan should haemorrhage occur.

1 **Attend to issues of consent**
- To administer blood in the face of refusal by a competent adult patient is unlawful.

2 **Reduce the risk of bleeding**
- Of particular importance to Jehovah's Witnesses, as replacement of haemorrhagic loss with bank blood is not an option.
- In the antenatal period treat anaemia and give attention to any complications which may predispose to bleeding.
- Senior staff should be involved in care so the best of skills are employed.
- Delivery should be managed routinely by experienced staff.
- Consultants should be sympathetic to the beliefs of Jehovah's Witnesses and plan care accordingly.
- If this is not the case, transfer care to another consultant.
- If there are no identified sympathetic consultants available contact the Hospital Liaison Committee for the names of sympathetic consultants.
- When the Jehovah' Witness goes into labour, inform the consultant obstetrician.
- If she needs a Caesarean section this should be carried out by a consultant.
- In the case of massive haemorrhage the consultant anaestheist and consultant haematologist should be involved.
- The advice of the consultant haematologist should be sought in the treatment of disseminated intravascular coagulation.
- Haemostasis must be meticulous.
- In the postpartum period, monitor for bleeding so early

intervention can be undertaken. Do not leave the patient alone for the first hour after delivery.

- Take care not to underestimate bleeding. Observe for signs of coagulopathy.
- After discharge from hospital the patient should have a lower threshold for seeking medical help for bleeding in the puerperium and should be given appropriate advice.
- Direct compression should be considered as a means of addressing bleeding.
- Give prophylactic oxytocics when the baby is delivered.

3 Stop blood loss

- If blood loss is stemmed early there is less risk of coagulopathy and therefore a reduced risk of further loss.
- Have a lower threshold for intervention – consider Caesarean hysterectomy at an earlier stage.
- Give haemabate or other oxytocins, ergometrine or prostaglandins for treatment of postpartum haemorrhage.
- Consider fibrinolytic inhibitors, e.g. tranexamic acid and aprotinin, cryoprecipitate, vitamin K, desmopressin.
- Cell salvage with leukocyte-depleting filters has been reported and may be considered

4 Optimize other physiological variables to reduce the effect of blood loss

- Give volume to treat hypovolaemia in the form of synthetic colloids and crystalloids.
- Use vasoconstrictors to maintain blood pressure.
- Give oxygen to optimize oxygen delivery.
- If very anaemic consider ventilation to optimize oxygen delivery.
- Start iron replacement and/or recombinant human erythropoietin.

CONSULT OTHER TOPICS

Caesarean hysterectomy (p. 52)
Consent (p. 183)
Massive obstetric haemorrhage – antepartum (p. 88)
Massive obstetric haemorrhage – DIC (p. 92)
Massive obstetric haemorrhage – postpartum (p. 95)
Risk management (p. 185)

SUPPLEMENTARY INFORMATION

Attend to issues of consent

There is variation amongst Witnesses as to which products and blood-saving techniques are acceptable. Obtain from the patient a clear statement of what she will accept and what she refuses.

Explain the risk of refusal of allogeneic blood frankly but not dramatically. Discuss earlier surgical intervention including the possibility of an earlier decision to proceed to Caesarean hysterectomy in uncontrolled postpartum haemorrhage. In the case of antepartum haemorrhage discuss with paediatrician the balance between delayed and immediate delivery and present these facts to the patient. If the patient continues to refuse blood products in the face of life-threatening haemorrhage proceed to Caesarean section.

If the mother is a minor, parental right to determine whether or not she will have medical treatment terminates if she has sufficient understanding and intelligence to enable her to comprehend fully what is proposed.

The wishes of a competent child may be overruled, if in the opinion of the court, the consequences of refusal are such that it would be inappropriate to comply with the child's wishes.

If the mother is too young to comprehend adequately and the parent refuses to agree to treatment that is in the opinion of qualified medical practitioners, proper and necessary, the matter can be referred to the High Court and this should be included in any case conferences. The High Court has emergency procedures to arrange for expedited considerations of such applications.

If the child is likely to succumb without the immediate administration of blood and the courts will be too time-consuming, blood should be transfused without consulting the court.

The patient and the parents must be kept informed of proposals.

Most Jehovah's Witnesses will carry with them a clear Advance Directive prohibiting blood transfusions and will have executed a Healthcare Advance Directive which gives comprehensive personal instructions on a variety of issues.

Healthcare Advanced Directives may be lodged with their GP as well as family and friends. If the patient is not in a condition to give or withhold consent, but has previously expressed a wish at an earlier date (Advance Directive or Healthcare Advance Directive), respect the patient's instructions in the Advance Directive or Healthcare Advance Directive, if that is applicable.

If such instructions do not specifically apply to the patient's current condition, or if the patient's instructions are vague and open to interpretation, or if there is good reason to believe that the patient has had a change of heart since making the declaration, the doctor's duty is to exercise good medical judgment and treat the patient in her best interests as determined by a responsible body of medical opinion.

Allow the patient the opportunity to speak with the Hospital Liaison Committee for Jehovah's Witnesses and if requested join their discussion.

Ensure that the patient has had the opportunity to speak with the obstetrician in privacy, without relatives or members of her religious community if she wishes.

Keep a clear record of discussion and particular aspects of consent. Note precisely which products/treatment she refuses and which she would accept. Complete a Jehovah's Witness consent form. Have discussion and take and document consent in the presence of a witness. The person witnessing the discussion should sign a record of the discussion and consent as made and signed by the doctor.

A verbally expressed change of mind should be honoured. Again it should be given in the presence of a witness and recorded in the notes.

Jehovah's Witnesses do accept reinfusion of their own blood when blood has not been stored and where equipment is arranged in a circuit which is constantly linked to the patients own circulatory system. Therefore the techniques of haemodilution, and blood salvaging, e.g. cell saver are acceptable.

Optimize other physiological variables to reduce the effect of blood loss

Cooling or hyperbaric environments can protect against the physiological effects of anaemia. These facilities are not in widespread use.

REFERENCES

The Hospital Liaison Committee for Jehovah's Witnesses. *Treating Jehovah's Witnesses in Obstetric and Gynaecology Departments.*

Association of Anaesthetists of Great Britain and Ireland (1999) *Management of Anaesthesia for Jehovah's Witnesses.*

Royal College of Surgeons of England (1996) *Code of Practice for the Surgical Management of Jehovah's Witnesses.*

USEFUL TELEPHONE NUMBERS

Hospital Information Services (Britain)   0181 906 2211

LOSS OF CONSCIOUSNESS OR FITTING

Level of consciousness is denoted by the Glasgow Coma Score (GCS).

Variable	Response	Score
Eye opening	Spontaneous	E 4
	To speech	3
	To pain	2
	Nil	1
Motor response	Obeys command	M 6
	Localizes pain	5
	Normal flexion to pain	4
	Abnormal flexion to pain	3
	Abnormal extension	2
	Nil	1
Verbal response	Orientated	V 5
	Confused	4
	Inappropriate	3
	Incomprehensible	2
	Nil	1

The highest score possible is 15.
The lowest score possible is 3.
A patient with a score of 8 or less is in a coma and requires to be intubated.
A fall in score of 2 or more points represents a significant deterioration in neurological condition.

ACTION PLAN

1 **If patient is fitting treat as eclampsia until proved otherwise**

2 **Call help including resident obstetrician and resident anaesthetist**

3 **Airway**
- Assess.
- Maintain patency.
- Apply oxygen 15 l/min via tight fitting face mask with reservoir bag.
- Call anaesthetist.
- Intubate.

Breathing
- Assess.
- Ventilate.

Circulation
- Assess pulse and BP.

- CPR.
- Put on ECG and NIBP monitor.
- Treat peri-arrest arrhythmias.
- Secure i.v. access, send blood for FBC, U&Es, LFTs, blood glucose, drug screen and cultures.
- Do immediate BMstix, start i.v.i.
- Treat hypotension.

4 **Place in left lateral position**

5 **Give i.v. dextrose if appropriate**

6 **Call anaesthetist to intubate if patient not already intubated and if gag reflex reduced or absent (GCS < 8)**

7 **Arrange ICU for intubated patient**

8 **Consider cause of unconsciousness/fit**

9 **Prevent secondary cerebral damage**

10 **Treat seizures with diazemuls 2.5–5 mg i.v. increments**

11 **Continuously monitor FH by cardiotocography if possible and consider timing and method of delivery**

12 **Keep record chart to include pulse BP, RR, SaO$_2$, GCS, U/O, FH and treatments given**

13 **Document event and treatment in notes, with time, date, a signature and printed identification and inform consultant obstetrician**

CONSULT OTHER TOPICS

SUPPLEMENTARY INFORMATION

Consider cause of unconsciousness/fit

- Eclampsia.
- Vasovagal.
- Hypotension.
- Local anaesthetic toxicity.
- Total spinal.

- Hyperventilation.
- Intracranial lesion.
- Any drug intoxication.
- Hypoglycaemia.

Call physicians, consider CT scan. If cause known start definitive treatment.

Prevent secondary cerebral damage

Keep well oxygenated, maintain BP, treat hypoglycaemia, treat seizures, restrict i.v. fluids if not hypovolaemic, head-up tilt if BP adequate and avoid constricting devices around the neck.

Treat seizures with diazemuls 2.5–5 mg i.v. increments

If still fitting after 10 mg i.v. summon anaesthetist as method of choice to control seizure is now thiopentone followed by intubation. If intubated ventilate to 4 kPA end tidal CO_2. In eclampsia magnesium 4 g 20% solution i.v. over 10 min can be used to treat the acute seizure. A maintenance infusion should be commenced to prevent recurrent seizure.

MAGNESIUM TOXICITY

C. Wasson

Magnesium sulphate is the drug of choice for seizure prophylaxis in pre-eclamptic patients. Its mechanism of action is mediated via NMDA receptors in the hippocampus and by antagonizing calcium-mediated cerebral vasoconstriction. The therapeutic plasma level is 2–4 mmol/l.

Magnesium sulphate has an extremely good safety record in pregnancy. It is vital, however, that the patient is monitored for signs of toxicity. If there is any suspicion, a plasma level should be checked.

Signs of toxicity are as follows

> 5 mmol/l	Loss of patellar reflexes
> 6 mmol/l	Generalized muscle weakness and respiratory difficulty
> 7 mmol/l	Paralysis of skeletal muscle and apnoea
> 10 mmol/l	Asystole

ACTION PLAN

1 **Stop administration of magnesium**

2 **Call for help including resident anaesthetist and obstetrician**

3 **Airway**
- Assess.
- Maintain patency.
- Apply oxygen 15 l/min via tight fitting face mask with reservoir bag.
- Attach pulse oximeter.

   Breathing
- Assess.
- Assist.
- Protect airway.

   Circulation
- Assess pulse and BP.
- CPR.
- Tilt to left.
- Put on ECG monitor.
- Treat peri-arrest arrhythmias.
- I.v. access, send bloods for FBC, U&Es, urgent plasma magnesium level.
- Treat hypotension.

4 **Give 10 ml of 10% calcium gluconate i.v. over 2–5 min if magnesium toxicity is likely**

5 **Do not give any further magnesium until plasma levels are known to be within or below the therapeutic range**

6 **Continuously monitor fetal heart by cardiotocography and consider timing and method of delivery**

7 **Keep record chart to include pulse, BP, RR, SaO$_2$, FH and treatments given**

8 **Record in notes and inform consultant obstetrician**

CONSULT OTHER TOPICS

Airway obstruction (p. 1)
Anaphylaxis (p. 133)
Cardiopulmonary resusciation (p. 8)
Peri-arrest arrhythmias (p. 16)
Respiratory emergencies (p. 20)
Spinals and epidurals – high spinal anaesthesia (p. 169)

SUPPLEMENTARY INFORMATION

Give 10 ml of 10% calcium gluconate i.v. over 2–5 min if magnesium toxicity is likely

Calcium antagonizes the action of magnesium at a cellular level. It is very effective in reversing the clinical effects of magnesium toxicity.

Do not give any further magnesium until plasma levels are known to be within or below the therapeutic range

Because magnesium is very effective in the prevention of eclamptic seizures, suspicion of toxicity should be confirmed by *immediate* biochemical analysis and where toxicity is excluded magnesium treatment can be restarted.

REFERENCE

Idama TO and Lindow SW (1998) Magnesium sulphate: a review of clinical pharmacology applied to obstetrics. *Br. J. Obstet. Gynaecol.* **105(3)**: 260–268.

Magnesium Toxicity

OLIGURIA AND ANURIA

Oliguria is defined as < 0.5 ml/kg/hour, anuria as < 100 ml/24 hours. Acute renal failure is suspected when oliguria persists despite adequate central venous and blood pressure.

1 **Consider causes of oliguria/anuria**

2 **Examine skin and CVS to assess volume status. Assess breathing, RR and SaO$_2$**

3 **Exclude or treat massive obstetric haemorrhage and pre-eclampsia**

4 **Insert urinary catheter**
- Measure residual volume and hourly urine output.
- Save urine for electrolytes and osmolality.

5 **Secure i.v. access with large bore cannula. Send bloods for FBC, U&Es. Group and save, coagulation studies and LFTs**

6 **Infuse 200 ml of colloid i.v. over 30 min**

7 **Monitor hourly urine output, half hourly pulse rate, blood pressure, RR and SaO$_2$**

8 **If urine output fails to respond to initial fluid bolus, i.e. less than 0.5 ml/kg/hour in the 30 min after the bolus given, give a second bolus of 200 ml of colloid**

9 **If no response to second fluid bolus consider CVP line**

10 **If fluid bolus inappropriate initially (because signs of fluid overload) consider CVP line**

11 **If pre-eclampsia excluded infuse colloid until CVP reading increases by 5 cmH$_2$O or up to 15 cmH$_2$O**

12 **When > 1 l colloid given, consider blood and blood products**

13 **If CVP > 15 cmH$_2$O consider acute renal failure**
- Call renal physicians.
- Consider ureteric obstruction if recent surgery.
- Recheck U&Es and arterial blood gases.

14 **Check fetal heart and consider timing and method of delivery**

15 **Keep record chart to include pulse, BP, CVP, RR, urine output, FH and treatments given**

16 **Document findings and treatment in notes, with time, date, a signature and printed identification**

CONSULT OTHER TOPICS

Caesarean section – complications (p. 55)
Eclampsia, pre-eclampsia, HELLP, fatty liver and hepatic rupture (p. 66)
Hypotension (p. 150)
Massive obstetric haemorrhage – antepartum (p. 88)
Massive obstetric haemorrhage – DIC (p. 92)
Massive obstetric haemorrhage – postpartum (p. 95)
Respiratory emergencies (p. 20)

SUPPLEMENTARY INFORMATION

Consider causes of oliguria/anuria

Most likely to be due to reduced renal perfusion secondary to hypovolaemia. Note recent surgery or pre-existing renal problems. Check notes for recent creatinine and urea levels. If history of renal problems contact renal physician.

The extent to which urine output is inadequate is a feature of how long the perfusion has been allowed to go untreated. There may, however, be early signs of acute renal failure where the cause is not decreased renal perfusion.

Other causes should be considered because the treatment for inadequate renal perfusion is fluid loading which, in itself, can be harmful in acute renal failure. A reason for the inadequate urine output should be sought early and used as a working diagnosis. It is beyond the scope of this text to provide a comprehensive list of causes. The commoner ones are as follows.

- Decreased renal perfusion.
- Intrinsic disease of the renal glomerulus as in chronic diabetes mellitus, polycystic kidneys, post-streptococcal infection.
- Intrinsic disease of the renal tubules as caused by toxins such as aminoglycosides, radiocontrast agents, myeloma protein or haemoglobinuria or by prolonged ischaemia.
- Intrinsic disease of the interstitium caused by pyelonephritis.
- Obstruction of ureters.

Pre-eclampsia, fatty liver, DIC and surgical ligation at Caesarean section are causes to be considered in pregnancy.

Investigations

Serum creatinine > 124 μmol/l and urea > 6.6 mmol/l are indicators of renal pathology.

Examine skin and CVS to assess volume status. Assess breathing, RR and SaO$_2$

Intravascular volume depletion

Early signs:

- Dry mouth.
- Loss of skin turgor.
- Cold peripheries.
- Increase in pulse rate.

Late signs:

- Further increase in pulse rate.
- Narrowing of pulse pressure.
- Fall in blood pressure.
- Increase in respiratory rate.
- Fall in level of consciousness.

If intravascular volume depletion is due to haemorrhage the patient may be pale.

Remember signs of pre-eclampsia and eclampsia.

Patient may be tachypnoeic or cyanosed due to pulmonary oedema or due to hypotension. If respiratory rate > 16/min or SaO_2 < 95% give oxygen 15 l/min via tight fitting face mask with reservoir bag.

Insert urinary catheter

If the patient already has a urinary catheter, irrigate the bladder. After placing the urinary catheter the residual volume of urine should be measured, recorded and compared to volume expected over time. Volume expected should be 0.5 × bodyweight × hours elapsed since last adequate volume voided (ml). Save urine in a sterile universal container for urine electrolytes and osmolality if later required.

When > 1 l colloid given, consider blood and blood products

Once the patient has been given replacement of 20% of their circulating blood volume as colloid, transfusion of blood should be considered. (Circulating blood volume = 100 ml/kg prepregnant weight.)

If CVP > 15 cm H$_2$O consider acute renal failure

If CVP and BP adequate but urine output remains inadequate the patient has acute renal failure. The condition is reversible but requires prompt and expert care in an HDU/ICU with renal support facilities.

SYSTEMATIC REVIEW

Offringa M (1998) Excess mortality after human albumin administration in critically ill patients. Clinical and pathophysiological evidence suggests albumin is harmful. *Br. Med. J.* **317**: 223–224.

SICKLE CELL CRISIS

E. Thomas and C. Cox

Sickling disorders include the heterozygous state sickle cell trait (HbAS), the homozygous sickle cell disease (HbSS) and compound heterozygous haemoglobin variants. The sickledex test confirms the presence of sickle haemoglobin (HbS) but does not quantify the amount, i.e. it detects trait, disease or variants but does not distinguish between them – haemoglobin electrophoresis is necessary for this. These states are most commonly seen in black people of African origin but may be seen in Saudi Arabians, Asians and people of Mediterranean origin. A low haemoglobin in the absence of bleeding in any of these populations may point to a diagnosis of sickle cell disease.

Sickle cell disease is a severe haemolytic anaemia. Patients with sickle cell disease suffer repeated painful crises due to the occlusion of the microvasculature by sickle cells.

Sickle cell crises are often precipitated by infection and exacerbated by dehydration, hypoxia, hypotension, hypothermia, acidosis and venous stasis. Sickle cell crisis is more common in pregnancy because of the hypercoagulable state.

ACTION PLAN

1 **Suspect**

2 **Inform senior obstetrician, anaesthetist, haematologist and paediatrician**

3 **Airway**
- Assess.
- Maintain patency.
- Apply oxygen 15 l/min via tight fitting face mask with reservoir bag.
- Attach pulse oximeter.
- Consider arterial blood gases.

   Breathing
- Assess.
- Ventilate.
- Protect airway.

   Circulation
- Assess pulse, BP and whether dehydrated.
- Put on ECG.
- Treat peri-arrest arrhythmias.
- Avoid frequent assessment of BP by inflation cuff if stable (venous stasis). If unstable consider arterial line.
- Secure i.v. access, send bloods for FBC, reticulocyte count, U&Es, LFTs, cross-match 4 units.

4 **Rehydrate**
- Ensure adequate hydration with Hartmann's or normal saline solution.
- Monitor fluid input and urine output.
- Avoid CVP line if possible.

5 **Consider need for transfusion**

6 **Monitor FH continuously by cardiotocography if viable and consider timing and method of delivery**

7 **Give adequate parenteral analgesia**
- Opiates i.v., i.m. or as patient controlled analgesia.

8 **Avoid hypothermia**

9 **Investigate cause**

10 **Treat crisis specifically**

11 **Keep a record chart to include pulse, BP, RR, SaO$_2$, FH and treatments given**

12 **Consider differential diagnosis**

13 **Organize haemoglobinopathy screening for baby, if appropriate**

14 **Document fully in notes with date, time, a signature and printed identification**

15 **Inform consultant obstetrician if not already aware**

CONSULT OTHER TOPICS

Acute abdominal pain (p. 44)
Acute chest pain (p. 128)
Cardiopulmonary resuscitation (p. 8)
Eclampsia, pre-eclampsia, HELLP, fatty liver and hepatic rupture (p. 66)
Hypotension (p. 150)
Intrauterine death (p. 81)
Jehovah's Witness patient (p. 153)
Massive obstetric haemorrhage – antepartum (p. 88)
Neonatal resuscitation (p. 14)
Peri-arrest arrhythmias (p. 16)
Premature labour (p. 110)
Respiratory emergencies (p. 20)

SUPPLEMENTARY INFORMATION

Consider need for transfusion

Advice must be taken from a consultant haematologist. *Simple 'top-up' transfusion* is used to maintain haemoglobin at a reasonable level (> 6 g/dl in sickle cell disease because well compensated for chronic anaemia) or to correct a rapid, significant fall (> 2–3 g/dl). Indications are as follows.

- Splenic or hepatic sequestration.
- Aplastic crisis (red cell aplasia due to parvovirus infection, etc.).
- Acute folate deficiency.
- Haemorrhage.

Exchange transfusion is used to reduce maternal haemoglobin to less than 30% to reduce the chance of sickling. Transfuse only to the normal haemoglobin level. Indications are as follows.

- Acute chest syndrome.
- Eclampsia and pre-eclampsia.
- Central nervous system involvement.

Monitor FH continuously by cardiotocography if viable and consider method and timing of delivery

Resuscitation of the mother should be carried out prior to the delivery of the baby.

Immediate delivery is not necessarily indicated if the CTG is non-reactive or the biophysical profile is unsatisfactory. Fetal parameters tend to improve and return to normal as the crisis improves.

Investigate cause

If temperature is raised, take blood for culture and commence antibiotics, augmentin or cefuroxime. A midstream specimen of urine (MSSU) and sputum sample should be taken as necessary. Request chest X-ray as indicated.

Treat crisis specifically

Painful crisis and acute hepatic or splenic sequestration are more common in the third trimester and postpartum period.

Painful crisis

(a) Presenting symptoms are fever, pain in the extremities, back, chest and abdomen.
(b) Clinical findings are tenderness over distal ends of long bones, lumbar spine, sternum and ribs, generalized abdominal tenderness, and dark urine.
(c) Investigations show evidence of disseminated intravascular coagulation (DIC), gamma glutamyl transferase (GGT) and total bilirubin raised. Magnetic resonance imaging (MRI) may show oedema and infarction of the bone marrow.
(d) Manage as above.

Acute hepatic or splenic sequestration

Common in HbSC and HbS β thallasaemia variants.

(a) Presenting symptoms are fever and abdominal pain and commonly bone pain.
(b) Clinical finding is progressive enlargement of the liver or spleen.
(c) Investigations – serial Hb estimations show a rapid fall to 30% of steady state Hb with a rise in reticulocyte count. Ultrasound will usually show enlargement of the liver and spleen. Gall stones and biliary tree obstruction should be looked for and excluded. Acute cholecystitis should be ruled out.
(d) Manage as above. If Hb is more than 2 g/dl below steady state give an immediate blood transfusion. Discuss with haematologist.

Aplastic crisis

(a) Presenting symptoms are pallor, fever, weakness and exertional dyspnoea.
(b) May show signs of high output cardiac failure.

Sickle Cell Crisis

(c) Investigations – serial Hb estimations show progressive anaemia to below 3.5 g/dl with a low reticulocyte count. Bone marrow aspirate shows giant pronormoblasts (hallmark of parvovirus infection).

(d) Management – transfuse to usual level of haemoglobin. Check serum folate level to rule out folate deficiency. Administer folic acid if low level. Spontaneous recovery can be expected in around 2 weeks.

Acute chest syndrome

(a) Presenting symptoms are fever, chest pain (pleuritic), shortness of breath and a non-productive cough.

(b) Clinical findings are signs of congestion, basal crepitations and signs of pleural effusion (diminished breath sounds and dullness at the bases).

(c) Investigations – chest X-ray shows patchy pulmonary infiltrations mainly in the lower lobes. Blood gases and lung scans show abnormalities.

(d) Manage as above, exclude pneumonia and pulmonary embolism, commence exchange transfusion, give broad spectrum antibiotics intravenously if the temperature is persistently above 38°C.

Avascular necrosis of the hip

(a) Presenting symptom is persistent hip pain made worse by walking and relieved by rest.

(b) Clinical findings are limited abduction with adduction deformity and apparent shortening of limb.

(c) Investigate by X-rays or MRI of the hip.

(d) Management – orthopaedic consultation, analgesia and non-weightbearing for 3–6 months.

Consider differential diagnosis

Conditions causing fever, pain and anaemia, e.g. acute febrile illnesses such as pneumonia or tonsillitis, obstetric problems such as pre-eclampsia and abruption, and surgical problems such as pyelonephritis, appendicitis, cholecystitis and pancreatitis and deep vein thromboses.

SYSTEMATIC REVIEW

Mahomed K (1999) Prophylactic versus selective blood transfusion for sickle cell anaemia during pregnancy (Cochrane Review). *The Cochrane Library*, Issue 2. Update Software, Oxford.

Reviewers' conclusions: *There is not enough evidence to draw conclusions about the prophylactic use of blood transfusion for sickle cell anaemia during pregnancy.*

SPINALS AND EPIDURALS – HIGH SPINAL ANAESTHESIA

C. Wasson

Suspect high spinal anaesthesia if a patient undergoing a spinal/epidural develops bradycardia, hypotension, tingling or weakness in the hands, or complains of difficulty with their breathing. Check level of sensation. If reduced sensation above the nipples this is a high spinal block.

A high spinal block is a local anaesthetic block involving the spinal nerves above the level of T4. It may occur due to excessive spread of a subarachnoid (spinal) injection of local anaesthetic (typically 2–3 ml of 0.5% bupivacaine) or following unintentional subarachnoid injection of an epidural dose of local anaesthetic (typically 10 ml of 0.25% or 0.5% bupivacaine).

Symptoms depend on the height of the block.

T1–T4	Bradycardia due to block of sympathetic cardiac nerves
C6–C8	Hand parasthesia and weakness
C3–C5	Diaphragmatic paralysis

Intracranial spread can also occur. It produces loss of consciousness due to the direct action of local anaesthesia on the brain. This is referred to as a 'total spinal'.

As with any spinal or epidural, peripheral vasodilatation due to block of the sympathetic nervous system (T1–L2) will lead to hypotension. This effect is exaggerated in a high spinal block and may produce sudden cardiovascular collapse.

ACTION PLAN

1 **Turn off epidural**

2 **Call for help including resident anaesthetist and obstetrician**

3 **Airway**
- Assess.
- Maintain patency.
- Apply oxygen 15 l/min via tight fitting face mask with reservoir bag.
- Attach pulse oximeter to patient.

Breathing
- Assess.
- Ventilate. Because of intercostal or diaphragmatic muscle paralysis the patient may complain of difficulty in breathing. If this compromises her ventilation she should be anaesthetized and intubated to assist ventilation until the effect of the local anaesthetic block wears off. If patient is apnoeic, intubate. If patient is hypoxic assist ventilation with face mask and self-inflating bag until anaesthetist arrives.
- Protect airway by intubation if patient is unconscious.

Circulation
- Assess pulse rate and BP.
- CPR.

- Tilt to left.
- Put on automatic BP and ECG monitor.
- Treat peri-arrest arrhythmias.
- i.v. access, send bloods for FBC, U&Es.
- Treat hypotension with i.v. colloids and ephedrine 3 mg increments titrated against BP.
- Treat bradycardia with atropine 0.6 mg i.v.

4 **Check fetal heart and consider timing and method of delivery**

5 **Consider and exclude other causes of unconsciousness**

6 **Keep record chart of pulse, BP, RR, SaO$_2$, FH and treatments given**

7 **Document in notes with time, date, a signature and printed identification and inform consultant anaesthetist and obstetrician**

CONSULT OTHER TOPICS

Airway obstruction (p. 1)
Cardiopulmonary resuscitation (p. 8)
Loss of consciousness or fitting (p. 157)
Peri-arrest arrhythmias (p. 16)
Respiratory emergencies (p. 20)
Spinals and epidurals – local anaesthetic toxicity (p. 171)

SUPPLEMENTARY INFORMATION

Consider and exclude other causes of unconsciousness

- e.g., hypoglycaemia, epilepsy, opioid drugs, intracranial lesion.

REFERENCES

Morgan B (1990) Unexpectedly extensive conduction blocks in obstetric epidural analgesia. *Anaesthesia* **45**: 148–152.

Scott DB and Hibbard BM (1990) Serious and fatal complications associated with extradural block in obstetric practice. *Anaesthesia* **64**: 537–541.

SPINALS AND EPIDURALS – LOCAL ANAESTHETIC TOXICITY

C. Wasson

Toxicity of local anaesthetics is due to their membrane stabilizing properties and mainly affects the brain and heart. It occurs following overdose by the intended route but more commonly due to inadvertent intravenous injection. Symptoms change with increasing plasma level:

Low dose	Tingling or numbness of tongue and perioral area
	Dizziness/tinnitus
	CNS irritability – twitching, anxiety, confusion
	Convulsions
	Loss of consciousness/respiratory depression
High dose	Cardiovascular depression and arrhythmias

ACTION PLAN

1 **Stop administration of local anaesthetics**

2 **Call for help including resident anaesthetist**

3 **Airway**
- Assess.
- Maintain patency.
- Apply oxygen 15 l/min.
- Attach pulse oximeter to patient.
- Consider intubation.

Breathing
- Assess.
- Ventilate.
- Protect airway.

Circulation
- Assess.
- CPR.
- Tilt to left.
- Put on ECG monitor.
- Treat peri-arrest arrhythmias.
- Treat hypotension with i.v. fluids and 3 mg bolus of ephedrine titrated against BP.
- i.v. access, send bloods for U&Es, start i.v.i.

4 **Control seizures**

5 **Check fetal heart and consider timing and method of delivery. Inform paediatrician**

6 **Keep record chart to include pulse, BP, RR, level of consciousness, FH and treatments given**

7 **Consider transfer to ICU**

8 **Document in notes, with time, date, a signature and printed identification and report to consultant obstetrician**

CONSULT OTHER TOPICS

Airway obstruction (p. 1)
Anaphylaxis (p. 133)
Cardiopulmonary resuscitation (p. 8)
Eclampsia, pre-eclampsia, HELLP, fatty liver and hepatic rupture (p. 66)
Loss of consciousness or fitting (p. 157)
Respiratory emergencies (p. 20)
Spinals and epidurals – high spinal anaesthesia (p. 169)

SUPPLEMENTARY INFORMATION

Airway and Breathing

Hypoxia rather than direct cardiovascular depression is the most common cause of cardiovascular collapse.

Circulation

Ventricular fibrillation and ventricular tachycardia are the most common arrhythmias. They are often resistant to electrical defibrillation. Bretylium is the antiarrhythmic drug of choice. Prolonged CPR may be required. Deliver the baby as a matter of urgency.

Control seizures

Diazepam 5–10 mg i.v. is the drug of choice. If this fails to quickly control seizures thiopentone followed by intubation and ventilation will be required. Ensure anaesthetist has been summoned.

REFERENCES

De la Coussaye JE and Eledjam JJ (1991) The pharmacology and toxicity of local anaesthetics. *Curr. Opin. Anaesthesiol.* **4**: 665–669.
Kasten GW and Martin ST (1985) Bupivacaine induced cardiovascular toxicity: comparison of treatment with bretylium and lidocaine. *Anaesthes. Analges.* **64**: 911–916.
Moore DC (1980) Administer oxygen first in the treatment of local anaesthesia-induced convulsions. *Anaesthesiology* **53**: 346–347.

SUBSTANCE ABUSE

E. O'Donnell, C. Wasson and K. Grady

Abuse refers to the use of a substance for recreational reasons. Substances which are abused include cannabis, opioid drugs, cocaine, amphetamines, benzodiazepines and, most commonly, alcohol.

Addiction is the compulsive continued use of a substance in spite of adverse consequences.

Dependence is the ability to develop a withdrawal reaction if the drug is not taken.

Tolerance is the requirement for increasing doses of a substance to achieve the same effect.

ACTION PLAN

1 **Identify substance abuse before or during pregnancy if possible**

2 **Initial presentation may be of an intoxicated patient – resuscitate**

In the most extreme cases this will require

Airway
- Assess.
- Maintain patency.
- Apply oxygen 15 l/min via tight fitting face mask with reservoir bag.
- Attach pulse oximeter to patient.
- Call anaesthetist.

Breathing
- Assess.
- Ventilate.
- Protect airway.

Circulation
- Assess pulse and BP.
- CPR.
- Tilt to left.
- Put on ECG and automatic BP monitor.
- Treat peri-arrest arrhythmias.
- Secure i.v. access, send bloods for FBC, U&Es, coagulation screen, drug screen, start i.v.i.
- Treat hypotension.

3 **Define a plan of substance intake during labour to prevent withdrawal, in discussion with senior obstetrician, psychiatrist, paediatrician and anaesthetist**

4 **Perform systemic review of cardiovascular, hepatic, renal and nutritional status**

5 **Screen for viral hepatitis, sexually transmitted disease and consider HIV screening**

6 **Closely observe mother during labour for signs of toxicity or withdrawal**

7 **Continuously monitor fetal heart by cardiotocography and consider timing and method of delivery**

8 **Review by consultant anaesthetist**
- Route of intravenous access.
- Methods of analgesia.
- Method of anaesthesia.

9 **Avoid contamination of staff or other patients by patient's body fluids**

10 **Inform paediatrician**

11 **After delivery**
- Discourage breastfeeding.
- Organize adequate contraception including barrier contraception.
- Offer counselling/drug rehabilitation.
- Organize multidisciplinary care.
- Undertake viral hepatitis, sexually transmitted disease, opportunistic cervical and HIV screening.

12 **Document in notes condition of patient and treatment provided with time, date, a signature and printed identification**

CONSULT OTHER TOPICS

Airway obstruction (p. 1)
Cardiopulmonary resuscitation (p. 8)
HIV and AIDS (p. 144)
Hypotension (p. 150)
Loss of consciousness and fitting (p. 157)
Neonatal resuscitation (p. 14)
Peri-arrest arrhythmias (p. 16)
Respiratory emergencies (p. 20)

SUPPLEMENTARY INFORMATION

Identify substance abuse before or during pregnancy if possible

This will allow for counselling, early screening for viral hepatitis, sexually transmitted disease and HIV and withdrawal and rehabilitation programmes. Consent and counselling must be provided for HIV screening.

Withdrawal without drugs but with inpatient support has been used. Barbiturates have also been used successfully. Benzodiazepines and disulfiram should be avoided in alcohol detoxification because of their potential teratogenicity.

Define a plan of substance intake during labour to prevent withdrawal in discussion with senior obstetrician, psychiatrist, paediatrician and anaesthetist

Oral methadone is used for the treatment of opioid addiction on the basis that it decreases intravenous use of illicit opioid drugs which carries greater risk to mother and baby. Regular methadone should be continued throughout delivery and postnatally to prevent withdrawal symptoms. If analgesia is required it must be provided by other means. Epidural local anaesthetic is advisable if there is no coagulopathy which would make the epidural injection contraindicated.

Symptomatic treatment of withdrawal should be planned in consultation with psychiatrists. Benzodiazepines are best avoided in the intrapartum period.

Perform systemic review of cardiovascular, hepatic, renal and nutritional status

Substance abuse is associated with many problems in both mother and fetus. The effects vary between substances.

Alcohol

Maternal cirrhosis, cardiomyopathy and pancreatitis and fetal alcohol syndrome.

Opioids

Maternal viral hepatitis, HIV, endocarditis and respiratory depression and intrauterine growth retardation.

Cocaine

Maternal myocardial ischaemia, arrhythmias, peripartum cardiomyopathy, convulsions, intracranial bleeding, renal and hepatic dysfunction and higher risk of fetal distress.

Amphetamines

Similar problems to cocaine.

Continuously monitor fetal heart by cardiotocography and consider timing and method of delivery

Placental insufficiency and intrauterine growth retardation are common. Therefore fetal distress is common and CTG monitoring is advised.

Review by consultant anaesthetist

Intravenous drug abuse may leave the mother with poor i.v. access. Central venous access may be necessary.

Opioid analgesia in standard doses is unlikely to be adequate in an opioid drug abuser.

Epidural analgesia should be considered but is contraindicated in the presence of a coagulopathy.

Avoid contamination of staff or other patients by patient's body fluids

Staff involved in the delivery should wear eye protection, protective waterproof clothing and double gloves. Extra caution should be taken to avoid needle stick injuries. Body fluids should be handled with care. Disposable instruments should be used where possible and fetal scalp electrodes or fetal blood sampling avoided where possible.

Inform paediatrician

Opioid withdrawal is common in the infant of an opioid abusing mother. The features include irritability with high pitched cry, respiratory distress, pyrexia, hypertonia and convulsions.

Naloxone administration may provoke a severe form of withdrawal syndrome. Oral methadone treatment in the mother can cause infant withdrawal.

After delivery

Breastfeeding should be discouraged as it may be associated with vertical transmission of HIV and hepatitis and the transfer of substances to the baby in breast milk.

The chosen contraceptive should not be user-dependent and should be coupled with a barrier method of contraception to protect against sexually transmitted diseases.

Children of drug addicted mothers have an increased risk of sudden infant death syndrome, developmental delay, and physical, emotional, and sexual abuse. For these reasons long-term paediatric and social service follow-up is required.

REFERENCE

Schubert PJ and Savage B (1995) Smoking, alcohol and drug abuse. In: James DK, Sneer PJ, Weiner CP and Gonik B (eds), *High Risk Pregnancy Management Options*. WB Saunders.

THROMBOEMBOLISM

The Report on Confidential Enquiries into Maternal Deaths in the United Kingdom 1994–1996 reports thromboembolism to be the leading cause of direct deaths. It recommends that there should be guidelines for thromboprophylaxis.

Pregnancy is a thrombogenic state in which the risk of deep vein thrombosis (DVT) is greatly increased.

ACTION PLAN

1 **Remember risk factors**

2 **Use antiembolism stockings until fully mobile and subcutaneous heparin in all high- and medium-risk women**

3 **Suspect pulmonary embolism**

4 **Call senior obstetrician, anaesthetist and medical team**

5 **Airway**
- Assess.
- Maintain patency.
- Apply oxygen 15 1/min via tight fitting face mask with reservoir bag.
- Attach pulse oximeter to patient.
- Consider early tracheal intubation if cardiovascular collapse or respiratory distress.

Breathing
- Assess.
- Ventilate with 100% oxygen if respiratory distress.
- May need positive end expiratory pressure to ventilate adquately.

Circulation
- Assess for signs of circulation and BP.
- CPR.
- Tilt to left.
- Put on ECG and BP monitor.
- Treat peri-arrest arrhythmias.
- Secure two large bore i.v. cannulae, send FBC, clotting studies and cross-match 6 units, run i.v.i.

6 **Request CXR, ECG and ABGs**

7 **If high probability, V/Q scan patient and anticoagulate**

8 **If the V/Q scan shows non high probability request pulmonary angiography**

9 **If positive diagnosis manage in intensive care unit, consider pulmonary artery flotation catheter (Swan Ganz) and continue supportive therapy**

CONSULT OTHER TOPICS

Airway obstruction (p. 1)
Cardiopulmonary resuscitation (p. 8)
Hypotension (p. 150)
Peri-arrest arrhythmias (p. 16)
Respiratory emergencies (p. 20)

SUPPLEMENTARY INFORMATION

Remember risk factors

- Caesarean section.
- Obesity.
- Other surgical procedures in pregnancy or puerperium.
- Congenital and acquired thrombophilia.
- Age – there is a 60-fold increase in risk over age 40 compared to age less than 25.
- Parity.
- Hypertensive problems.
- Prolonged labour.
- Instrumental delivery.
- Confined to bed.

Use antiembolism stockings until fully mobile and subcutaneous heparin in all high- and medium-risk women

Heparin 5000 iu (or 20 mg for enoxaparin) 12 hourly if medium-risk or 8 hourly if high-risk.

Suspect pulmonary embolism

May present as cardiovascular collapse or pulmonary oedema, sudden shortness of breath, tachypnoea and pleuritic chest pain. There may be hypotension with raised jugular venous pressure and hypoxia.

If high probability, V/Q scan patient and anticoagulate

Start heparin and maintain APTT 1.5–2.5 control value. Urgent V/Q scan. A normal V/Q scan conclusively excludes a pulmonary embolism.

TRANSFUSION REACTIONS

Allogeneic blood transfusions (transfusion of blood from another individual) can result in transfusion reactions, anaphylactic or allergic responses or infection.

Acute transfusion reactions can be:	• Haemolytic
	• Non-haemolytic
Haemolytic reactions can be:	• Intravascular (almost always due to transfusion of ABO incompatible blood)
	• Extravascular (due to other antibodies)

ACTION PLAN

1 **During transfusion**
- Observe for first 15 min.
- Monitor temperature at 0, 15 and 30 min and then hourly from the start of each unit.
- Monitor pulse at 0, 15 and 30 min and then hourly.
- Monitor blood pressure at the beginning and halfway through the unit (if no indication to measure it more regularly).

2 **Suspect haemolytic transfusion reaction if pain in arms, loin or chest, dyspnoea, flushing or chills**

3 **Stop transfusion**
- Quickly check for ABO incompatibility. If ABO compatible continue emergency management of symptoms. Tell blood bank immediately as unit of blood intended for your patient could be transfused to another patient.

4 **Call for help including resident anaesthetist and inform haematologist**

5 **Airway**
- Assess.
- Maintain patency.
- Apply oxygen 15 l/min via tight fitting face mask with reservoir bag.
- Attach pulse oximeter to patient.

Breathing
- Assess.
- Ventilate.
- Protect airway.

Circulation
- Assess pulse and BP.
- CPR.
- Tilt to left.
- Put on ECG monitor.
- Treat peri-arrest arrythmmias.
- I.v. access, send bloods for FBC, direct antiglobulin test (same tube), U&Es, LFTs, clotting studies, blood cultures and send 5 ml in dry tube for repeat compatibility testing.
- Treat hypotension.

6 **Consider anaphylaxis**

7 **Run normal saline 100–200 ml i.v.**

8 **Catheterize bladder and record urine output every 15 min**

9 **Give fluids to maintain urine output > 1.5 ml/kg/hour**

10 **Consider need for CVP line**

11 **Give frusemide/furosemide 80–120 mg i.v.**
- if urine output < 1.5 ml/kg/hour and CVP > 0 cmH$_2$O and patient not hypotensive.

12 **Give mannitol 20% 100 ml**
- if no diuresis after frusemide/furosemide.

13 **Assume acute renal failure and obtain specialist help**
- if urine output 2 hours after mannitol and frusemide/furosemide is < 1.5 ml/kg/hour.

14 **Adjust infusion rate to maintain urine flow > 1.5 ml/kg/hour**

15 **Call renal physicians if hyperkalaemic and check arterial blood gases to exclude acidosis**

16 **Repeat FBC, U&Es and coagulation screen 2–4 hourly. Send to blood bank remainder of blood unit and transfusion giving set**

17 **Contact consultant haematologist if coagulopathy**

18 **Contact consultant haematologist if patient needs further transfusion**

19 **Double check the labelling on the unit of blood with patient's identification band and with other identifiers**
- Confirm or exclude haemolytic reaction.

20 **Late pyrexia or rigors in the absence of other signs is probably due to a non-haemolytic reaction**
- Stop transfusion, send sample and blood unit to blood bank and give aspirin 0.6–0.9 g p.o. Observe closely until symptoms and signs resolve. Discuss further transfusion with haematologist.

21 **Urticaria and itching at the start of transfusion in the absence of other signs are probably due to an allergic reaction**
- Give chlorpheniramine 4 mg p.o. and stop transfusion for 30 min. If urticaria and itching resolve restart transfusion.

22 **For any reaction keep record chart of pulse, BP, RR, SaO$_2$, temperature, FH and treatments given**

23 **Check fetal heart and continuously monitor by cardiotocography**
- In severe haemolytic reaction consider appropriate timing of delivery.

24 **Record reaction in notes chronologically with date, a signature and printed identification and inform and explain to patient**

25 **Report serious adverse events following transfusion to Serious Hazards of Transfusion (SHOT) Group**

CONSULT OTHER TOPICS

Airway obstruction (p. 1)
Anaphylaxis (p. 133)
Cardiopulmonary resuscitation (p. 8)
Hypotension (p. 150)
Oliguria and anuria (p. 162)
Respiratory emergencies (p. 20)

SUPPLEMENTARY INFORMATION

Suspect haemolytic transfusion reaction if pain in arms, loin or chest, dyspnoea, flushing or chills

Intravascular haemolytic reactions are rare but have a high mortality from disseminated intravascular coagulation (DIC) and acute renal failure (ARF). They occur during the first few ml of transfusion and are characterized by pain in the arms, loins and chest, hypotension and red urine. Group A blood into a Group O patient causes the most severe reaction.

Extravascular haemolytic reactions can cause an immediate, severe reaction if transfusion is rapid or a delayed reaction. Immediate severe reactions may lead to ARF.

Stop transfusion

Although haemolytic transfusion reaction is rare it can be fatal. Symptoms and signs appear after 5–10 ml. Prognosis is much worse if 200 ml or more have been given. Transfusion should be stopped as soon as a reaction is suspected.

Consider anaphylaxis

Very rarely severe anaphylaxis can occur (due to antibodies to IgA). Signs of anaphylaxis are angio-oedema, laryngeal oedema, bronchospasm, hypotension and cardiovascular collapse.

Run normal saline 100–200 ml i.v.

To maintain renal blood flow to prevent ARF. Hyperkalaemia and metabolic acidosis are signs of ARF.

Repeat FBC, U&Es and coagulation screen 2–4 hourly. Send to blood bank remainder of blood unit and transfusion giving set

Transfusion giving set is examined to exclude bacterial contamination as a cause of transfusion reaction.

Double check the labelling on the unit of blood with patient's identification band and with other identifiers

Direct antiglobulin test confirms a haemolytic reaction.

Late pyrexia or rigors in the absence of other signs is probably due to a non-haemolytic reaction

Non-haemolytic reactions are commonly called febrile reactions (due to white cell antibodies). They occur in approx. 1% of transfusions and are characterized by fever or rigors 30–60 min after the start of the transfusion.

Urticaria and itching at the start of transfusion in the absence of other signs are probably due to an allergic reaction

They are insignificant if there is no progression of symptoms after 30 min cessation of transfusion. Give chlorpheniramine 4 mg p.o. and stop transfusion for 30 min. If urticaria and itching resolve restart transfusion.

REFERENCE

Blood Transfusion Services of the United Kingdom (1996) *Handbook of Transfusion Medicine*. Her Majesty's Stationery Office, London.

USEFUL TELEPHONE NUMBER

Serious Hazards of Transfusion (SHOT) Group   0161 273 7181

Transfusion Reactions

CONSENT

Informed consent means that the patient has all the necessary information to make a decision regarding their submission to a procedure. It should not be confused with written consent which is a permanent record that a conversation took place and is not legally binding.

Failure to obtain informed consent may give rise to civil or criminal proceedings as any touching of the person no matter how well intentioned is a trespass.

CONSENT FOR MINORS

- The United Nations Convention on Rights of the Child and the Children Act 1989 establish the child's right to be consulted.
- The Gillick principle states that 'the child's full consent is required if the child is of sufficient understanding to make an informed decision, which is for the doctor to decide'.
- The above is open to interpretation and makes no distinction between the giving and refusing of consent and tacitly acknowledges that children mature at different rates.
- Children can only truly consent if they understand the nature, purpose and hazards of the treatment.
- Consent should be obtained from the child's parent or guardian.
- Jehovah's witnesses – for children under the age of 16 without capacity to consent the doctors duty is to the patient and he or she may give blood or blood products if they are a necessary component of the relevant treatment, regardless of parental wishes. (High Court permission may be needed.)
- A parental refusal of advance consent to an operation considered necessary to the child's health may be challenged in the High Court.

CONSENT TO CAESAREAN SECTION

- Most Caesarean sections are carried out for fetal reasons, usually fetal distress. However the mother's life may be at risk, e.g. from fulminating pre-eclampsia, obstructed labour or placenta praevia.
- In law the fetus has no rights. An unborn child is not a separate person from its mother. The mother therefore cannot be forced to submit to an invasion of her body against her will, e.g. be subjected to a Caesarean section.
- A woman detained under the Mental Health Act cannot be forced into medical procedures unconnected with her medical condition unless her capacity to consent to such treatment is diminished.
- The pregnant woman is entitled to make decisions which put her life or her baby's life at risk as long as she is adjudged to be mentally competent.

| ACTION PLAN | 1 | Have full discussion with the pregnant woman and her partner, family or friends with regard to the perceived risk of the decision taken by the pregnant woman. The discussion should be documented and witnessed |

ACTION PLAN

1 Have full discussion with the pregnant woman and her partner, family or friends with regard to the perceived risk of the decision taken by the pregnant woman. The discussion should be documented and witnessed

2 Senior medical staff should be consulted, i.e. the relevant consultants from the involved specialities

3 The hospital legal advisor should be consulted and a decision taken whether the woman has mental capacity and whether an application should be made to the courts to detain the woman under The Mental Health Act 1983

CONSULT OTHER TOPICS

Jehovah's Witness patient (p. 153)
Risk management (p. 185)

REFERENCES

Seeking patients' consent: the ethical considerations. General Medical Council.
Panting GP (1998) *Consent*. Medical Protection Society.

USEFUL TELEPHONE NUMBERS

General Medical Council	0171 580 7642
Medical Defence Union	0171 935 5503
	0161 491 3301
Medical Protection Society	0171 399 1300
	0113 243 6436
Medical and Dental Defence Union of Scotland	0141 221 5858

Consent

RISK MANAGEMENT

Risk management is an essential part of good obstetric and midwifery practice. It has been made essential by increased litigation against Trusts, doctors, nurses and midwives. Medical staff of all grades should belong to a medical defence organization.

ACTION PLAN

1 **ALWAYS keep clear records which are timed, dated and signed with your name printed underneath**
- Remember good notes equal good defence, poor notes equal poor defence and no notes equal no defence.

2 **ALWAYS record clearly drug prescriptions, intravenous infusion prescriptions and allergies**

3 **ALWAYS be meticulous in writing up operative notes**
- Record the station as well as the position of the head abdominally as this is as equally important at Caesarean section as it is at instrumental vaginal delivery.

4 **ALWAYS be honest**
- If there were difficulties with delivery of the baby document them and record manoeuvres performed with timings.

5 **ALWAYS ask for senior assistance if you suspect injury to other structures and record this in the notes**

6 **ALWAYS, if you suspect that an incident may become the subject of a complaint, obtain contemporaneous statements from witnesses and discuss them with the consultant obstetrician and the clinical risk manager**
- Have a high index of suspicion. If you suspect a potentially litigious situation record the events but do not place this record in the notes. Keep a copy yourself and forward one to your risk manager.

7 **ALWAYS get informed consent, e.g. risk of Caesarean hysterectomy if operating for postpartum haemorrhage**

8 **ALWAYS record patient refusal to comply with suggested treatment and have it witnessed**

9 **ALWAYS tell the truth**

10 **NEVER alter the records**
- Even if grossly inaccurate or libellous. Write a revised version with timings, dates and signature with printed name underneath.

11 **NEVER under any circumstances erase or delete any part of the record**
- This includes cardiotocographs.

12 **NEVER criticize a medical, nursing or midwifery colleague in front of a patient or the patient's relatives and never enter criticisms into the notes**
  - If concerned about a colleague's performance discuss this with the clinical/medical director.

13 **NEVER record any personal remarks or derogatory comments about the patient or her relatives in the notes**
  - However, records should be kept in the notes of aggressive behaviour, bad language, threats and evidence of intoxication or substance abuse.

14 **NEVER delegate inappropriately**

CONSULT OTHER TOPICS

Consent (p. 183)

SUPPLEMENTARY INFORMATION

- There has been a rapid increase in legal actions relating to midwifery care.
- The reasons for this include an increased expectation which has been encouraged by government – The Patients' Charter – coupled with resource limitation and so-called cost improvement.
- Complaints are encouraged – they are jewels to be treasured!
- There is now a strong blame culture – 'it must be someone's fault'.
- Many problems arise from poor communication, with lack of formal handovers contributing to this.
- Inadequate supervision contributes to obstetric medical litigation.
- Fear of litigation paradoxically often leads to worse care.
- Doctors may not be able to rely on their employers to look after their interests and should therefore retain membership of a medical defence organization.

USEFUL TELEPHONE NUMBERS

Medical Defence Union	0171 935 5503
	0161 491 3301
Medical Protection Society	0171 399 1300
	0113 243 6436
Medical and Dental Defence Union of Scotland	0141 221 5858

APPENDIX I

Guidelines for the control of blood glucose during labour in insulin-treated women

1 *To be used for spontaneous labour, induction of labour and elective Caesarean section unless* insulin has been given within the last 4 hours or baseline blood glucose > 17 mmol/l.

(a) Measure blood glucose on arrival and hourly thereafter using BMstix and/or reflectance meter.

(b) Commence glucose/potassium/insulin (GKI) infusion as follows:

10% dextrose 500 ml
Potassium chloride 10 mmol } 8 hourly, i.e. approx 60 ml/hour
Actrapid insulin as per glucose

(c)	If blood glucose	< 2.0	mmol/l	No insulin – dextrose only
	If blood glucose	2.1–4.0	mmol/l	Add 8 units insulin
	If blood glucose	4.1–9.0	mmol/l	Add 16 units insulin
	If blood glucose	9.1–11.0	mmol/l	Add 24 units insulin
	If blood glucose	11.1–16.9	mmol/l	Add 32 units insulin

(d) Aim for target of 4–9 mmol/l. Keep infusion rate constant at 500 ml 8 hourly but change insulin concentration in a new bag of dextrose according to blood glucose.

(e) If blood glucose < 2 mmol/l give 10% dextrose only and check BMstix every 30 min until > 4 mmol/l and then start GKI as above.

(f) If blood glucose > 17 mmol/l set up low-dose insulin infusion at 3 units/hour until < 11 mmol/l for 2 hours.

(g) Just prior to delivery make a new 500 ml bag of 10% dextrose plus 10 mmol KCl plus half the amount of insulin in the current infusion bag.

(h) Start this new solution as quickly as possible after delivery. Use a new giving set flushed through with the new concentration of insulin.

(i) Once patient is able to eat and drink give insulin in a dose similar to that used before pregnancy 20 min before their next meal and take GKI down 1 hour later.

2 **To be used when insulin *has* been given in the last 4 hours**

(a) Determine blood glucose as before.

(b) If blood glucose:	> 11.1	mmol/l	Treat as above
	4.1–11.0	mmol/l	Add 12 units insulin to GKI
	< 4.0	mmol/l	10% Dextrose only

(c) Commence routine once blood glucose > 4 mmol/l.

3 **To be used if blood glucose > 17 mmol/l at outset**

(a) Make up low-dose insulin infusion of 50 units actrapid insulin in 50 ml normal saline and infuse at 3 units/hour (3 ml/hour).

(b) When blood glucose < 11mmol/l for 2 consecutive hours set up conventional GKI regimen as above.

SUPPLEMENTARY INFORMATION

- Patients often need less insulin overnight.
- Patients should not have a full meal on a GKI regimen but light snacks and beverages are allowed.
- The GKI regimen provides 1.5 l of water over 24 hours and may cause hyponatraemia, particularly if simultaneous syntocinon infusion.
- Insulin has an i.v. half-life of about 5 min so any prolonged interruption of transfusion will result in rebound hyperglycaemia.

APPENDIX II
RELEVANT DOCUMENTS
AND ENQUIRIES
Why mothers die

The Confidential Enquiries into Maternal Deaths in the United Kingdom 1994–1996 showed that 376 women died in this period giving a maternal mortality rate of 12.2 per 100 000 maternities. There were 134 direct deaths, 134 indirect deaths, 36 fortuitous deaths and 72 late deaths.

Of the 134 direct deaths, 48 were due to thromboembolism, 20 due to pregnancy-induced hypertension, 19 due to amniotic fluid embolism, 15 due to early pregnancy complications (12 ectopic pregnancies) and 14 to sepsis. The above five causes account for 85% of maternal deaths.

Haemorrhage accounted for 12 deaths, uterine rupture for three, fatty liver of pregnancy for two and anaesthesia for one.

There were 134 indirect deaths: 39 were due to cardiac disease, 19 to epilepsy and nine to psychiatric causes.

Recommendations were made for auditable standards for maternity care. It was recommended that each unit should have a lead clinician responsible for guidelines and that guidelines should be in place for the management of pre-eclampsia and eclampsia, the management of obstetric haemorrhage, the use of thromboprophylaxis, the use of antibiotics for Caesarean section, the management of women who decline blood products, and the identification and management of ectopic pregnancy.

Importantly, it was recommended that units should organize 'fire drills' for the management of obstetric emergencies and that training should be provided in the recognition of domestic violence, post natal depression and the correct use of car seat belts.

REFERENCE

Confidential Enquiries into Maternal Deaths 1994–96. HMSO, London.

Confidential Enquiry into Stillbirths and Deaths in Infancy (CESDI)

CESDI is under the umbrella of the National Institute for Clinical Excellence (NICE). The remit is to encourage effective practices to be implemented and for harmful practices to be minimized.

STILLBIRTHS

Stillbirths form 35% of all losses. 'Unexplained' and 'unavoidable' are terms often used, but in 45% of cases there were potential avoidable factors.

The majority of fetal deaths occur in low risk women.

Post-mortem modified the clinical assessment in 15% of cases.

INTRAPARTUM DEATHS

Intrapartum deaths represent 15% of deaths.

Avoidable factors during labour were identified in 72%.

Babies weighing 4 kg or more are significantly less likely to die than smaller babies during pregnancy and up to the first year of life. However, these large babies are significantly more likely to die intrapartum.

ANTENATAL CARE

Failure to recognise or deal with a suspected large baby is the most common antenatal factor.

INTRAPARTUM CARE

The most common problem with intrapartum care was inaccurate interpretation of the CTG. Delay in delivery and inappropriate choice of the mode of delivery was the second most common problem. For example, with a clinically suspected large baby the possibility of shoulder dystocia should be considered and experienced staff should be available. There should be clear protocols for the management of shoulder dystocia and 'fire drills' should be practised.

RECORD KEEPING

Poor record keeping occurs in a third of cases.

REFERENCE

Confidential Enquiry into Stillbirths and Deaths in Infancy, Sixth Annual Report, 1999.

Towards safer childbirth

The recommendations from the 'Towards Safer Childbirth' document are as follows.

1.1 The organization of labour wards should be reviewed and improved, and if necessary changes implemented to reflect the recommendation in this report.

1.2 All labour wards should have a lead consultant obstetrician and clinical midwife manager.

1.3 The lead obstetrician will be responsible for day to day management, staff deployment, training and support of medical staff. The clinical midwife manager will have parallel responsibilities for midwifery personnel.

1.4 There should be a multidisciplinary labour ward forum comprising, at a minimum, the lead obstetrician, the clinical midwife manager, an obstetric anaesthetist, a neonatal paediatrician, a risk manager, representatives from junior medical and midwifery staff and a consumer representative from the Maternity Services Liaison Committee to review labour ward activity and develop guidelines.

1.5 There should be a set of referenced, evidence-based guidelines which should be dated, signed and reviewed on a regular basis, every one to three years. Past guidelines and protocols should be dated and archived in case they are needed for reference at a later date.

1.6 The documentation and storage of data should be rigorous and precise. The use of computerized documentation, using recognised and acceptable programmes, should be encouraged.

1.7 Staffing, both medical and midwifery, should be in line with the following standards.

- At a minimum consultant or equivalent cover should be available in a supervisory capacity for 40 hours during the working week, unless the unit is small and where the majority of women who give birth have had a normal pregnancy.
- Junior staffing levels will depend on available training opportunities.
- Midwifery staffing levels should be in line with those recommended by the Audit Commission, namely 1.15 midwives per woman in labour.
- There should be a clinical midwife leader available on each shift.

1.8 Midwives and medical staff should be able to communicate and consult freely and at an appropriate level.

1.9 The consultant on-call from the labour ward should conduct labour ward rounds at least twice during the day with a telephone or physical round during the evening.

1.10 In the case of emergencies, anticipated difficult deliveries or whenever a woman's condition gives rise to anxiety, the consultant on the labour ward should be contacted.

1.11 Six-monthly multidisciplinary in-service education/training sessions on the management of 'high risk' labours and CTG interpretation should be attended by all clinicians. A log book of attendances should be kept.

1.12 The outcome measures and standards described should be adopted and audited annually in line with best practice.

REFERENCE

Towards Safer Childbirth, Minimum Standards fro the Organisation of Labour Wards, Report of a Joint Working Party. February 1999.

Appendix II

INDEX

Index

NORMAL VALUES

...ernal arterial blood gases

Parameter	Range
pH	7.4–7.45 ('alkalosis' of pregnancy)
PaO_2	13.9–14.4 kPa (104–108 mmHg)
	Same as non-pregnant for age
$PaCO_2$	3.6–4.3 kPa (27–32 mmHg)
	Non-pregnant value 4.4–6.1 kPa (33–46 mmHg)
Bicarbonate	18–31 mmol/l
	Non-pregnant value 22–26 mmol/l

Cord blood

Parameter	Arterial	Venous
Mean pH	7.24–7.28	7.32–7.36
Mean $PaCO_2$	5.9–7.5 kPa	5.1–5.3 kPa
Mean base excess	6.8–7.7 mmol/l	3.5–6.1 mmol/l
PaO_2	6.7–12 kPa	
Bicarbonate		18–31 mmol/l